Diabetes

Paleo Diet Recipes for Diabetics

By

Barbara P. Trisler

Copyright ©2017

All rights reserved. Except as permitted under the U.S. Copyright Act of 1976, the scanning, uploading and distribution of this book via the Internet or via any other means without the express permission of the author is illegal and punishable by law. Please purchase only authorized electronic editions, and do not participate in or encourage electronic piracy of copyrighted material.

Disclaimer

This publication is designed to provide competent and reliable information regarding the subject matter covered. However, it is sold with the understanding that the author is not engaged in rendering medical or other professional advice. Laws and practices often vary from state to state and country to country and if medical or other expert assistance is required, the services of a professional should be sought. The author specifically disclaims any liability that is incurred from the use or application of the contents of this book.

Table of Contents

Introduction..9

Chapter 1 – Understanding Diabetes...12

- Type 1 Diabetes..13
- Type 2 Diabetes..13
- Gestational Diabetes..14

Chapter 2 – What is the Paleo Diet?..16

Chapter 3 – The Benefits of the Paleo Diet for Diabetics....................18

Chapter 4 – Paleo Diet Foods to Eat and Avoid..................................22

- Foods to Eat on the Paleo Diet..23
- Foods to Avoid on the Paleo Diet..26

Chapter 5 – Tips for Getting Started on the Paleo Diet.......................27

Chapter 6 – Paleo Diet Recipes for Diabetics.....................................30

- Breakfast Recipes..33
  - Blueberry Coconut Smoothie...34
  - Tomato Basil Omelet..36
  - Spiced Apple Walnut Muffins..38
  - Ham and Red Pepper Frittata..40
  - Pumpkin Pie Pancakes..42
  - Strawberry Ginger Beet Smoothie...44
  - Pumpkin Pecan Muffins..55
  - Creamy Avocado Walnut Smoothie...57

4

- Vegetable Egg White Omelet..59
- Cinnamon Coconut Flour Waffles..60
- Triple Berry Smoothie..62
- Mixed Vegetable Frittata...63
- Sweet Apple Pancakes..65
- Blueberry Muffins..67
- Almond Butter Banana Smoothie.......................................69

○ Lunch Recipes...70
- Curried Butternut Squash Soup..71
- Avocado Egg Salad..73
- Roasted Tomato Basil Soup...74
- Avocado Spinach Salad with Egg..76
- Creamy Sweet Potato Soup..78
- Apple Walnut Chicken Salad...80
- Hearty Beef and vegetable Stew..81
- Balsamic Strawberry Kale Salad..83
- Cream of Broccoli Soup..84
- Mushroom and Leek Soup...87
- Creamy Cucumber Dill Salad..89
- Lamb and Root Vegetable Stew...91
- Mango Walnut Salad with Pecans......................................92
- Easy Chicken and Vegetable Soup......................................94

○ Dinner Recipes..98

- Rosemary Roasted Chicken..99
- Thai Coconut vegetable Curry..101
- Herb-Roasted Pork Tenderloin...103
- Balsamic Grilled Salmon..105
- Slow Cooker Pulled Pork...107
- Veggie-Stuffed Zucchini Boats...109
- Baked Haddock with mango Salsa......................................111
- Seared Scallops with Herb Butter.......................................113
- Meatloaf with BBQ Sauce...114
- Herb-Crusted Lamb Chops...116
- Slow Cooker Chicken Cacciatore..118
- Zucchini Pasta and Meatballs...120
- Chicken Tikka Masala...122
- Sausage Sweet Potato Chili...124
- Cajun Chicken and Veggies..128
- Easy Garlic Shrimp...130
- Bacon-Wrapped Turkey Breast...132
- Grilled Salmon with Mango Sauce......................................133
- Lemon Chicken with Broccoli..135
- Maple BBQ Ribs...137
- Cilantro Lime Chicken...139
- Curry Grilled Pork Chops..141

- Snacks and Dessert...142

- Baked Cinnamon Apple Chips..................................143
- Avocado Deviled Eggs..................................145
- Easy Coconut Flour Cupcakes..................................146
- Vanilla Almond Trail Mix..................................148
- Chocolate Chia Pudding..................................149
- Choco-Coconut Cupcakes..................................151
- Sesame Kale Chips..................................153
- Almond Butter Brownies..................................155
- Cinnamon Roasted Nuts..................................156
- Almond Flour Apple Crisp..................................158
- Coconut Date bites..................................160
- Lemon Blueberry Cupcakes..................................162
- Grilled Balsamic Peaches..................................163
- Maple Walnut Trail Mix..................................165
- Cinnamon Poached Pears..................................166
- Coconut Almond Chia Pudding..................................168
- Baked Beet Chips..................................169
- Cranberry Coconut Trail Mix..................................171

- Bonus: Paleo Diabetic Protein Shakes..................................172
  - Vanilla Almond Protein Shakes..................................174
  - Chocolate Strawberry Protein Shake..................................176
  - Cinnamon Banana Protein Shake..................................177
  - Tropical Peach Protein Shake..................................179

- Mocha Almond Protein Shake..................................180
- Choco-Banana Coconut Protein Shake.....................182
- Apple Pie Protein Shake..183
- Brownie Batter Protein Shake...................................184
- Almond Coconut Protein Shake................................186
- Coconut Cream Pie Protein Shake............................188
- Spiced Chai Protein Shake..189
- Matcha Protein Shake...191

Conclusion...192

Introduction

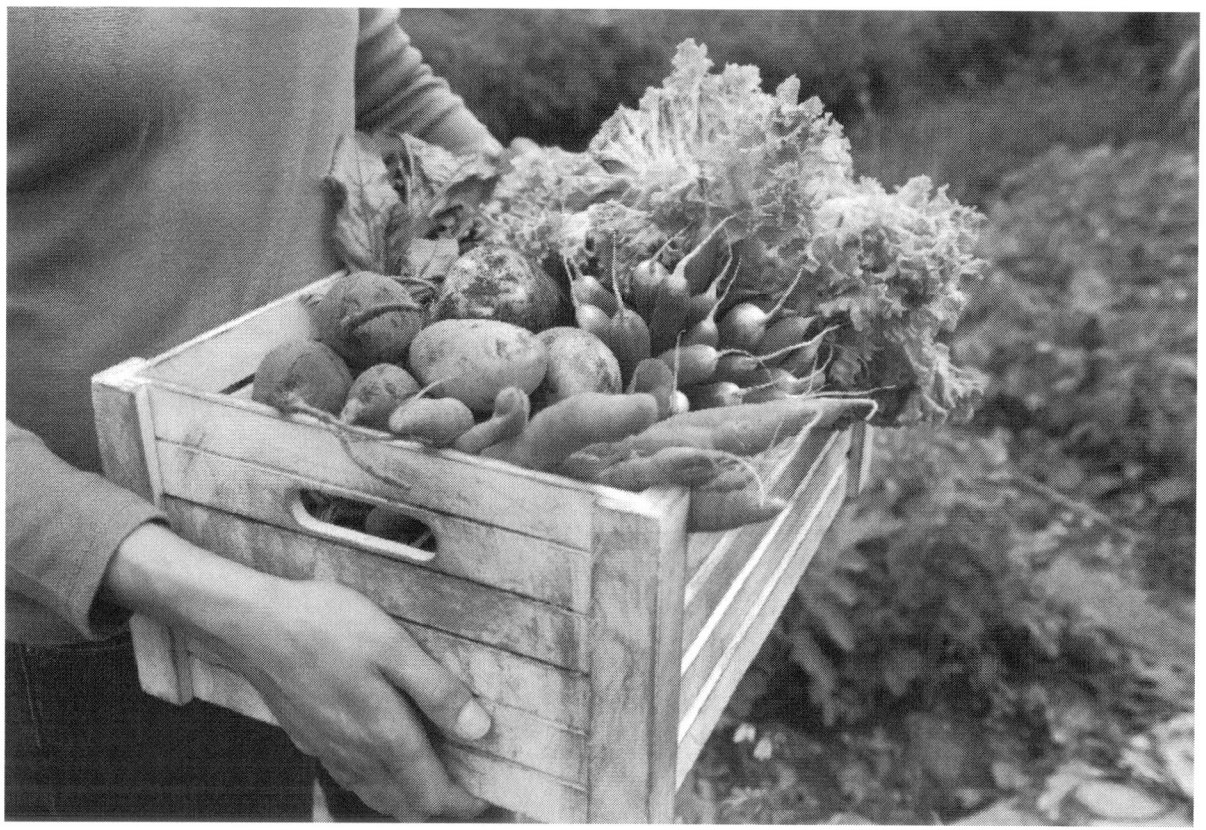

All it takes is a quick glance at the magazine rack at your local grocery store to keep up with the latest fad diets. These days it seems like a new diet hits the shelves every week, always making lofty promises of weight loss and improved health. Unfortunately, many of these diets are not based on a foundation of scientific truth and any results they produce fade quickly. While many diets are not worthy of your consideration, there is one that is – the paleo diet. Whether you want to lose weight, improve your digestion, or boost your overall health, this is the diet to try.

Some people know of the paleo diet as the caveman diet because it is based on the type of diet our Paleolithic Era ancestors followed. Though you don't have to hunt or scavenge for food, you do need to adhere to certain rules if you're going to follow the paleo diet. This diet excludes processed carbs and refined sugars as well as dairy products, grains, and legumes. It might sound a little restrictive at first but, once you get used to it, you'll be free from the negative health effects caused by the average Western diet and you'll be feeling better than you ever have before.

The paleo diet is scientifically proven to provide a wide range of health benefits. If you're reading this book, there is one benefit you are probably most interested – reversing diabetes. Type 2 diabetes affects millions of people, many of which do not make even the slightest effort to control or reverse their condition. With a healthy diet and regular exercise, however, it is entirely possible to reverse this condition! The paleo diet is a diet that is typically *high in lean protein and fiber but low in carbohydrates and fat* – exactly the type of diet that will help you stabilize your blood sugar, improve your insulin sensitivity, and manage your diabetes.

For many, diabetes is a lifelong condition. With the help of the paleo diet, however, it is possible to *reverse* type 2 diabetes and manage type 1 diabetes, reducing your dependence on supplemental insulin. If you'd like to learn more about the paleo diet and its benefits for diabetes, simply turn the page and keep reading!

Chapter 1

Diabetes Type 1 and 2

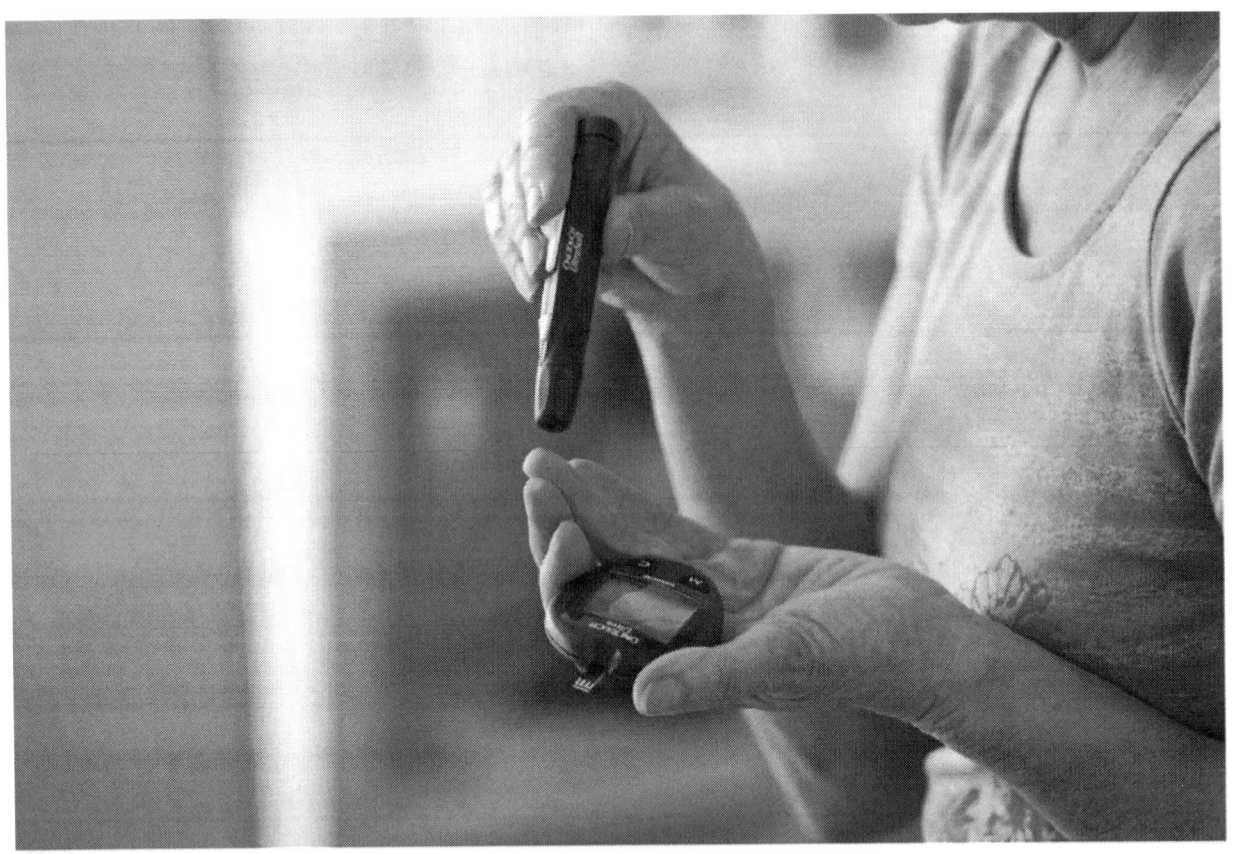

All of the food you eat contains nutrients like protein, carbohydrates, and fat. Each of these nutrients plays an important role in your total health and wellness and they also contain energy. Most of the food you eat can be broken down into glucose by your digestive system. From there, a hormone called insulin helps your body absorb and utilize that glucose as a source of energy. Insulin is produced in the pancreas and your production of insulin varies depending on the type of food you're eating and how easy it is to digest. Foods that digest quickly (simple carbohydrates like white rice or bread) have a greater impact on your blood glucose levels than foods that take longer to digest (complex carbohydrates like whole grains).

When you eat, the insulin produced by the pancreas helps to transport the glucose from food to your bloodstream then to your cells where it can be used as energy. If you eat too many foods that cause your blood sugar level to spike and to remain high, your body might become resistant to the effects of insulin – it will take more and more insulin to produce the desired effect. High blood sugar is the defining characteristic of diabetes, though there are several different types of diabetes. Here is a quick overview of each:

Type 1 Diabetes

This type of diabetes is an autoimmune condition in which the immune system accidentally attacks healthy cells in the pancreas, preventing it from producing insulin. This condition is usually diagnosed in childhood or early adolescence and it typically requires lifelong treatment with insulin.

Type 2 Diabetes

This type of diabetes is acquired and it can develop at any age. Type 2 diabetes typically develops when the body becomes resistant to the effects of insulin or if insulin production becomes impaired. This type of diabetes is particularly common in people who are overweight or obese and it can often be *reversed* if the patient improves his or her lifestyle.

Gestational Diabetes

This type of diabetes is seen in pregnant women and it often goes away after the baby is born. Having gestation diabetes increases your risk for developing type 2 diabetes later in life and sometimes type 2 is incorrectly diagnosed as gestational diabetes.

Diabetes affects nearly 30 million people in the United States – that's more than 9% of the American population. What's more, as many as 1 in 4 people who have diabetes don't even know it. In addition to obesity, other risk factors for diabetes include physical inactivity, family history of diabetes, race, high blood pressure, and other health problems. Treatment for diabetes generally involves taking supplemental insulin, though making healthy changes to your lifestyle can be beneficial as well.

When left untreated, diabetes can lead to some very serious complications including heart disease, kidney disease, nerve damage, eye problems, and stroke. Having diabetes can also reduce circulation to the extremities which, in some cases, leads to serious infections that eventually require amputation of the affected limb. Though there are differences between type 1 and type 2 diabetes, the symptoms of both are similar and may include:

- Excessive thirst
- Increased urination

- Extreme hunger
- Ketones in the urine
- Unexplained weight loss
- Fatigue
- Blurry vision
- Irritability
- Slow-healing of wound and sores
- Frequent infections

Diabetes can be a lifelong condition, though type 2 can potentially be reversed by making healthy lifestyle changes. For many people, losing weight by increasing physical activity and improving diet helps to reverse diabetes, though insulin treatments may still be needed while these changes are being put into effect. The best diet for someone with diabetes is a *high-protein, high-fiber diet that is low in processed carbohydrates and moderate in healthy fats.* Though you can certainly make these dietary changes on your own, many people find that the paleo diet works to improve their condition. You'll learn more about the paleo diet in the next chapter.

Chapter 2

What is the Paleo Diet?

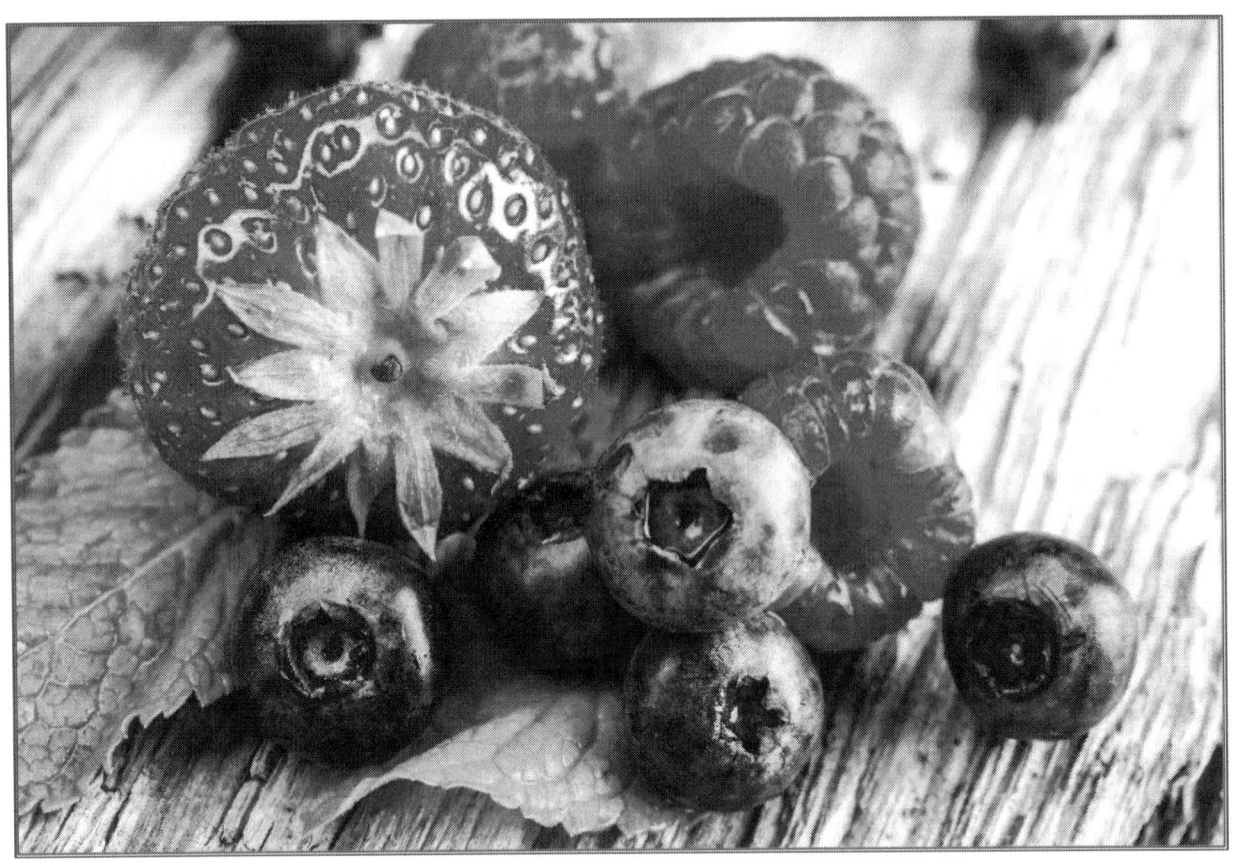

There are countless fad diets out there that promise amazing results but many of them don't actually work or, if they do, the results are short-lived. The paleo diet is more than just a fad diet – it is a healthy lifestyle that involves eating wholesome, natural foods that have been largely unaltered by man. The name paleo diet comes from the Paleolithic Era when humans lived hunter-gatherer lifestyles. Agriculture had not yet been developed, so humans lived off the land, hunting game and gathering other edibles. The modern paleo diet is based on the idea that human genetics have not changed significantly since the

Paleolithic Era and, therefore, humans are still biologically optimized for a diet made up of natural foods.

Following the paleo diet doesn't require you to hunt for your own food, but it does require you to think a little more carefully about your dietary choices. This diet is *focused primarily on lean proteins, fresh fruits and vegetables, nuts, seeds, and healthy fats.* The paleo diet excludes all processed foods and refined carbohydrates as well as dairy products, grains, and legumes. Essentially, the paleo diet includes foods that would have been available to our Paleolithic Era ancestors prior to the birth of agriculture. There is some wiggle room, of course, but that is the leading principle behind the diet. In the next chapter, you'll learn about the benefits of the diet.

Chapter 3

The Benefits of the Paleo Diet for Diabetics

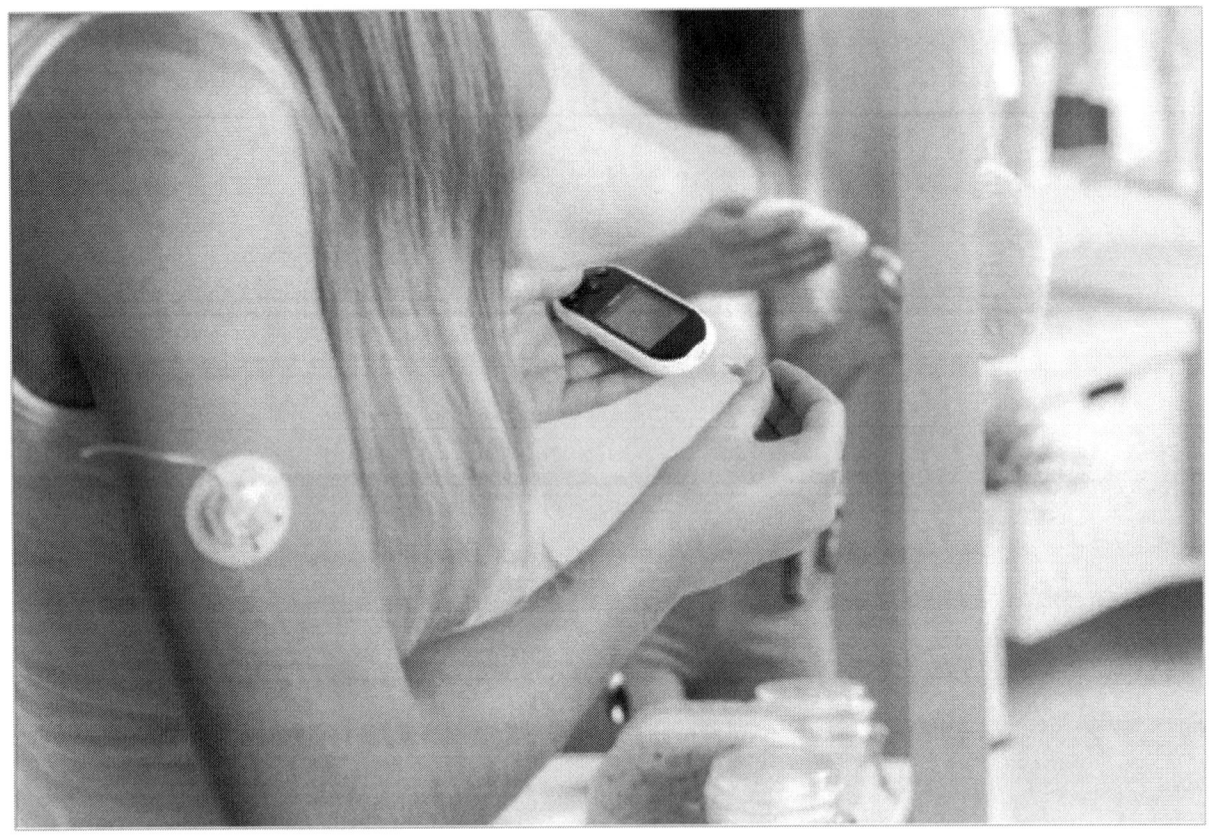

The paleo diet is focused around wholesome, natural foods like lean meats and seafood, fresh fruits and vegetables, nuts, seeds, and healthy fats. As such, the paleo diet overlaps with aspects of certain other diets that have been linked to significant health benefits including the Mediterranean diet and the DASH diet. Though many would call the paleo diet restrictive, it is actually much simpler to follow than you might think. You must cut out grains and dairy products, but that still leaves you with plenty of options. We'll go into greater detail about the foods that you can and can't eat on the paleo diet in a later chapter – for now, let's focus on the benefits of the paleo diet.

The benefits of the paleo diet are similar to the benefits of any diet that is developed around wholesome, natural foods. Here are some of the top benefits:

a) More lean muscle mass:

The paleo diet is focused on lean proteins like grass-fed meat, free-run poultry, and wild-caught fish – all of these help you to build and maintain lean muscle mass.

b) Improved digestive health:

Refined sugars and processed carbohydrates can cause inflammation in the intestinal tract which can impair your body's ability to properly digest and utilize nutrition from the foods you eat. Removing these foods will allow your digestive system to heal.

c) Increased longevity:

Following a diet low in processed foods and saturated fat has been shown to increase lifespan – it also helps you to avoid chronic diseases which might shorten your lifespan.

d) Highly concentrated nutrition:

The foods that are included in the paleo diet are naturally rich in nutrients – synthetic vitamins and minerals used to fortify processed foods are less biologically valuable than natural sources for the same nutrients.

e) **Fewer allergies:**

The paleo diet is naturally free from some of the most common food allergens such as grains like corn and wheat – it is also free from dairy products.

f) **Reduced inflammation:**

Chronic inflammation is a leading factor behind numerous diseases including cardiovascular disease. Many of the foods included in the paleo diet have anti-inflammatory benefits.

g) **Increased energy levels:**

When you cut out foods that damage your digestive system and interfere with the absorption of nutrients, your body can begin to heal. As your digestion improves and you start absorbing nutrients once more, your energy levels will improve as well.

h) **Healthy weight loss:**

Though the paleo diet isn't strictly low-calorie, many of the foods included are nutrient-dense and lower in calories than most processed foods. This diet can help you lose weight and keep it off.

i) Reduced risk for disease:

Many of the most serious chronic diseases are, at least in part, related to an unhealthy diet. Improving your diet can help to reduce your risk for serious diseases.

In addition to the benefits already listed, the paleo diet is also particularly beneficial for people with diabetes. By removing refined sugar and processed carbohydrates from your diet, you can stabilize your blood glucose levels to avoid blood sugar spikes. Once your blood sugar stabilizes, your body can begin to repair and heal itself from insulin resistance, enabling you to once more digest and absorb nutrition from the food you eat. The paleo diet can also help you to achieve and maintain a healthy bodyweight which will help you to prevent your diabetes from coming back once you successfully reverse it. Keep reading to learn about the specifics of the paleo diet.

Chapter 4

Paleo Diet Foods to Eat and Avoid

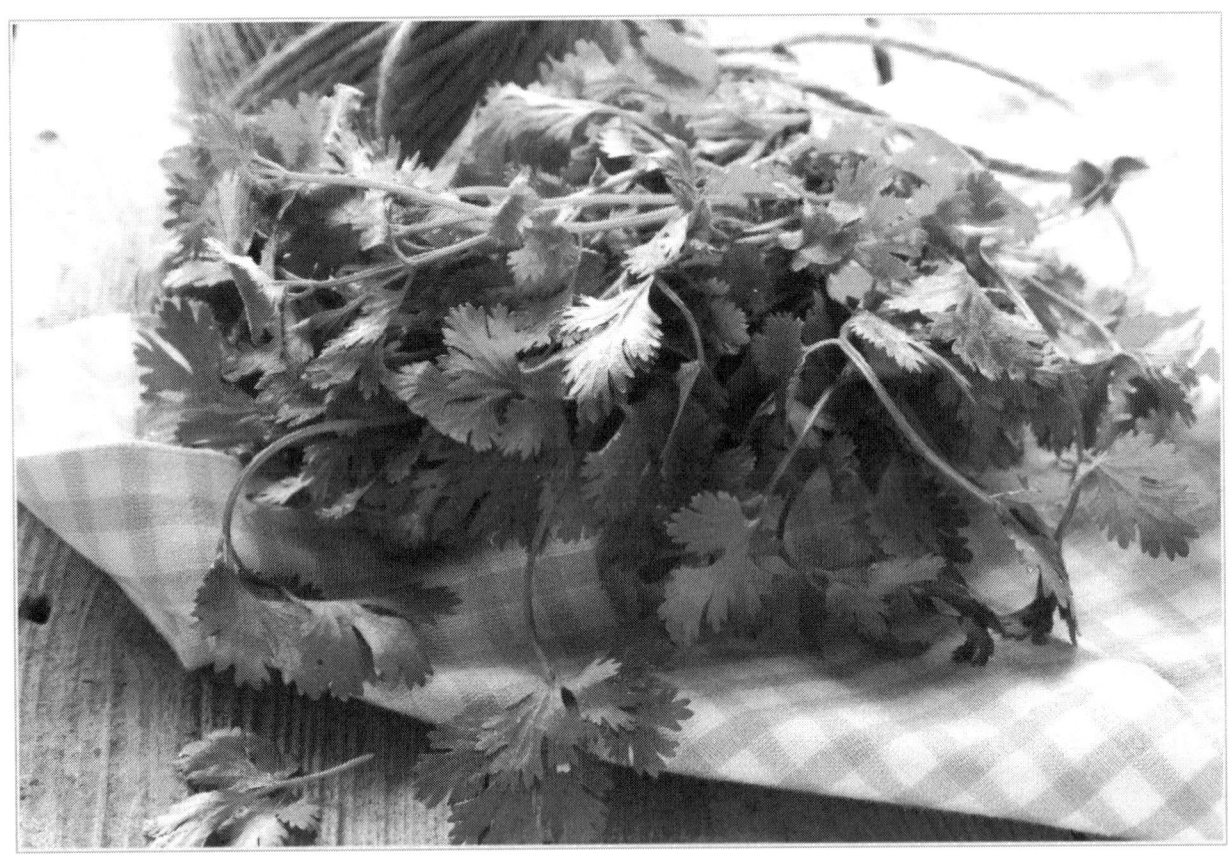

As you have already learned, the paleo diet is made up of wholesome, natural foods – foods that have been minimally altered by man. This includes lean proteins like grass-fed meats, free-run poultry, cage-free eggs, and wild-caught fish as well as fruits and vegetables. It also includes nuts, seeds, and healthy fats. Refined sugars and processed carbohydrates have no place in the paleo diet, nor do dairy products, grains, legumes, or potatoes. To help you see exactly which foods are and are not allowed on the paleo diet, here are some helpful food lists:

Foods to Eat on the Paleo Diet

Proteins		
Bacon	Chicken	Eggs
Beef	Clams	Elk
Bison	Duck	Fish
Goose	Pork	Shrimp
Lamb	Quail	Turkey
Lobster	Rabbit	Veal
Pheasant	Scallops	Venison

Fruits & Vegetables		
Apples	Cherries	Onions
Apricots	Cucumber	Papaya
Asparagus	Eggplant	Parsnips
Artichoke	Grapes	Peaches
Arugula	Grapefruit	Pears
Bananas	Green beans	Pineapple
Beets	Guava	Plum
Bell peppers	Herbs	Pomegranate
Bok choy	Honeydew	Pumpkin
Blackberries	Kale	Raspberries

Blueberries	Kohlrabi	Spinach
Broccoli	Kiwi	Strawberries
Brussels Sprouts	Lemon	Sweet potato
	Lime	Swiss chard
Cabbage	Lettuce	Squash
Carrots	Leeks	Tomatoes
Cantaloupe	Mango	Turnips
Cauliflower	Mushrooms	Watermelon
Celery	Nectarines	Zucchini

Nuts & Seeds		
Almonds	Brazil nuts	Cashews
Chestnuts	Macadamia nuts	Sesame seeds
Chia seeds	Pecans	Walnuts
Flaxseeds	Pine nuts	Hazelnuts
Hemp seeds	Pumpkin seeds	Turkey

Healthy fats		
Avocados	Macadamia oil	Coconut oil
Olive oil	Ghee	Tallow

| Grass-fed butter | Lard | Walnut oil |

Other Foods		
Almond flour	Dark chocolate	Honey
Almond milk	Arrowroot powder	Maple syrup
Baking powder	Pepper	Salt
Baking soda	Cocoa powder	Spices
Coconut	Stevia	Coconut aminos
Tapioca starch	Coconut flour	Tea
Coconut milk	Vanilla extract	Coffee
Vinegar		

Foods to Avoid on the Paleo Diet

Fruits & Vegetables		
Alcohol	Frozen yogurt	Artificial sweetners
Ice cream	Baked goods	Lentils
Barley	Margarine	Beans
Oats	Bread	Pasta
Brown rice	Peanuts	Brown sugar
Peanut butter	Candy	Potatoes
Canola oil	Quinoa	Cereal
Rye	Cheese	Soft drinks
Chickpeas	Soy beans	Corn
Soy sauce	Cornstarch	Split peas
Corn oil	Vegetable oil	Couscous
Wheat	Cow's milk	White rice
Cream cheese	White sugar	Energy drinks
Yogurt		

N/B: This list is by no means complete but it gives you an idea what foods to look out for. Avoid all grains, dairy products, and legumes as well as processed foods and refined sugars.

Chapter 5

Tips for Getting Started on the Paleo Diet

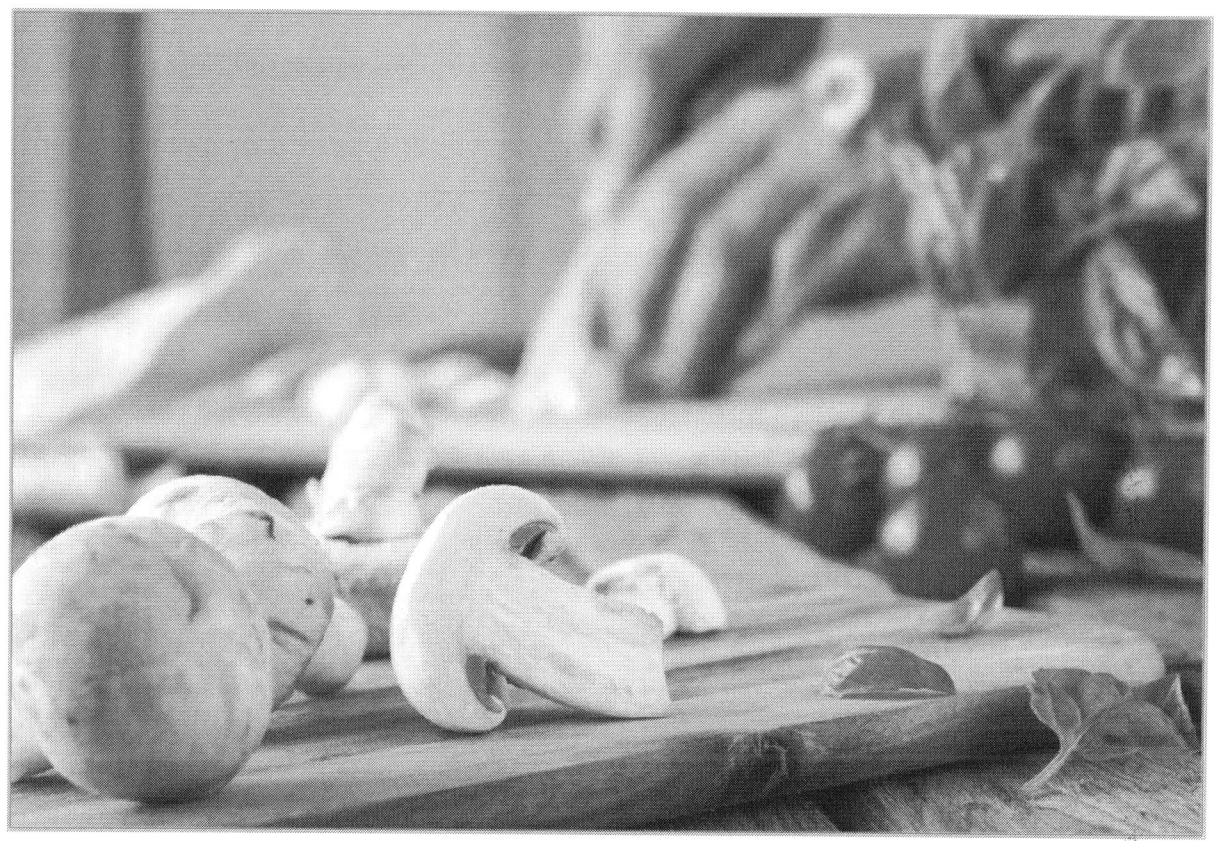

The paleo diet is more a lifestyle than an actual diet – it incorporates certain dietary principles but also advocates for a healthy lifestyle in general. If you'd like to give the diet a try, there are some simple things you can do to ease yourself through the transition – here are some tips:

- Start increasing your protein intake and reducing your carbohydrate intake – you should also be eating a moderate amount of healthy fats.
- Swap fresh fruits and vegetables for grains and legumes – be sure to include some vegetables at every meal.

- Replace hydrogenated oils with coconut oil or olive oil for cooking and limit your intake of saturated fats.
- Stop using refined sugars like granulated sugar and brown sugar, swapping in natural sweeteners like honey and pure maple syrup.
- Focus on healthy cooking methods like grilling, baking, broiling, and poaching instead of frying.

As you make these changes to your diet, you'll find that adhering to the principles of the paleo diet is not as difficult as you once imagined. When shopping for groceries, take the paleo food list from the previous chapter with you so you know what to look for. Generally speaking, however, most of the foods you find in the outer aisles at the grocery store are safe – things like fresh produce, meat, and seafood. If you're going to commit to the paleo diet, you might want to start by cleaning out your pantry of all non-paleo foods and then stock up on approved foods so you have plenty of options.

Just because you're following the paleo diet doesn't mean that you can't enjoy food. Fresh herbs and dried spices are all included in the diet and can be used to add flavor to your favorite paleo dishes. You can also continue to eat out while following the paleo diet, though you might have to order different dishes than you're used to. Dishes that feature grilled meats, salads, and many other entrees are already made with paleo-friendly ingredients or they can be made paleo with some minor adjustments. If you don't see something on the menu that fits the paleo diet, you can always order a green salad with grilled chicken or fish.

As you transition into the paleo diet, you may experience some withdrawal symptoms that result from cutting grains out of your diet. Fortunately, these symptoms usually only last a few days for most people. During this time, be sure to drink plenty of water and make sure to get adequate rest as well. It is also a good idea to make small changes over time instead of going cold-turkey on everything. The more gradually you make changes to your diet and lifestyle, the more they will become a habit and the easier those changes will be to maintain.

Chapter 6

Paleo Diet Recipes for Diabetics

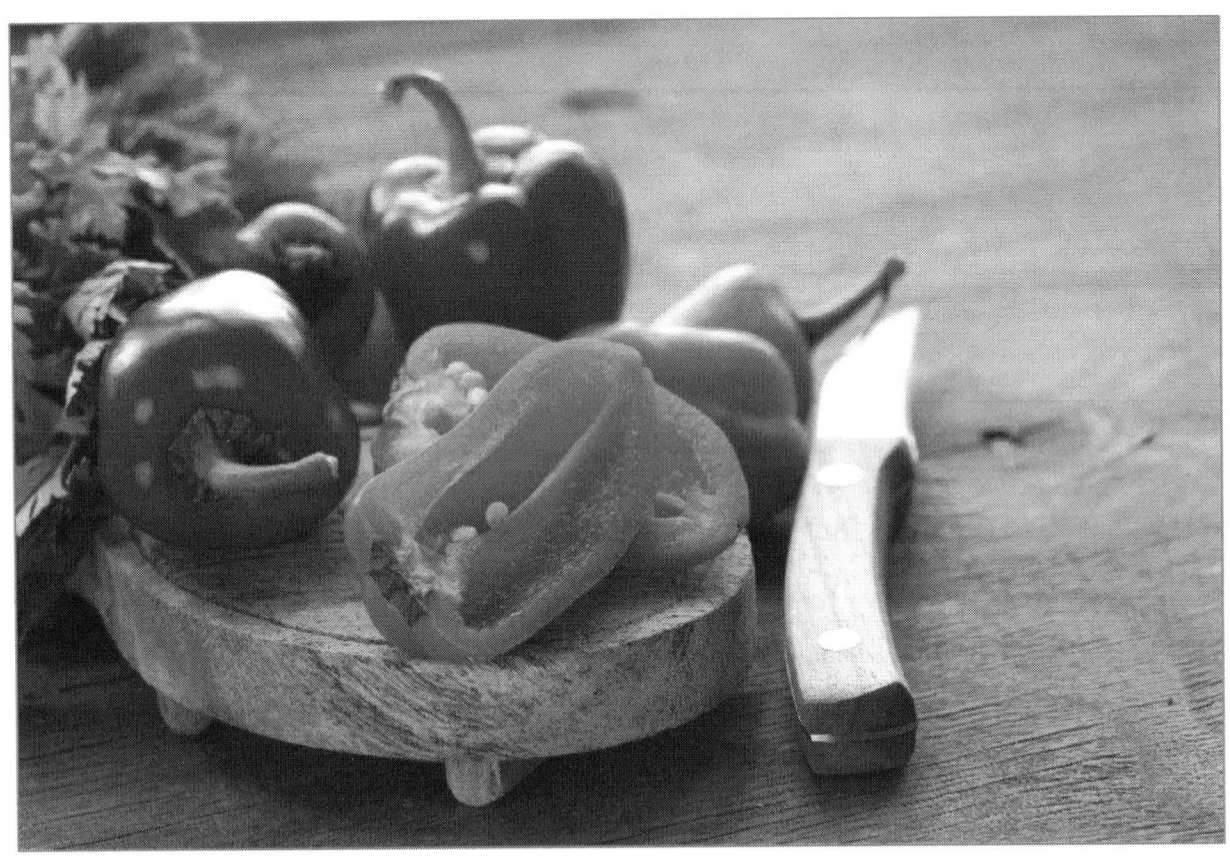

Now that you have a better understanding of the paleo diet and which foods are and are not included, you're ready to give it a try for yourself! In this chapter, you'll find a collection of delicious paleo recipes for breakfast, lunch, dinner, snacks, and dessert.

Recipes Included in this book

1	Blueberry Coconut Smoothie	2	Coco-Vanilla Chia Pudding
3	Tomato Basil Omelet	4	Spinach and Mushroom Omelet

5	Spiced Apple Walnut Muffins	6	Cinnamon Banana Pancakes
7	Ham and Red Pepper Frittata	8	Raspberry Kale Smoothie
9	Pumpkin Pie Pancakes	10	Pumpkin Pecan Muffins
11	Sweet Potato Breakfast Skillet	12	Vegetable Egg White Omelet
13	Strawberry Ginger Beet Smoothie	14	Cinnamon Coconut Flour Waffles
15	Triple Berry Smoothie	16	Thai Cocunut Vegetable Curry
17	Mixed Vegetable Frittata	18	Herb-Roasted Pork Tenderloin
19	Sweet Apple Pancakes	20	Balsamic Grilled Salmon
21	Blueberry Muffins	22	Veggie-Stuffed Salmon
23	Almond Butter Banana Smoothie	24	Slow Cooker Pulled Pork
25	Curried Butternut Squash Soup	26	Baked Haddock with Mango Salsa
27	Avocado Egg Salad	28	Meatloaf with BBQ Sauce
29	Roasted Tomato Basil Soup	30	Seared Scallops with Herb Butter
31	Avocado Spinach Salad with Egg	32	Herb-Crusted Lamb Chops
33	Creamy Sweet Potato Soup	34	Zucchini Pasta and Meatballs
35	Apple Walnut Chicken Salad	36	Slow Cooker Chicken Cacciatore
37	Hearty Beef and Vegetable Stew	38	Chicken Tikka Masala
39	Balsamic Strawberry Kale Salad	40	Sausage Sweet Potato Chili
41	Cream of Broccoli Soup	42	Slow Cooker Balsamic Roast Beef
43	Chopped Chicken and Mango Salad	44	Cajun Chicken and Veggies
45	Mushroom and Leek Soup	46	Easy Garlic Shrimp

47	Creamy Cucumber Dill Salad	48	Bacon-Wrapped Turkey Breast
49	Lamb and Root Vegetable Stew	50	Grilled Salmon with Mango Sauce
51	Mango Walnut Salad with Pecans	52	Lemon Chicken with Broccoli
53	Easy Chicken and Vegetable Soup	54	Maple BBQ Ribs
55	Spiced Pumpkin Soup	56	Cilantro Lime Chicken
57	Rosemary Roasted Chicken	58	Curry Grilled Pork Chops
59	Baked Cinnamon Apple Chips	60	Almond Flour Apple Crisp
61	Avocado Deviled Eggs	62	Coconut Date Bites
63	Easy Coconut Flour Cupcakes	64	Lemon Blueberry Cupcakes
65	Vanilla Almond Trail Mix	66	Grilled Balsamic Peaches
67	Chocolate Chia Pudding	68	Maple Walnut Trail Mix
69	Choco-Coconut Cupcakes	70	Cinnamon Poached Pears
71	Sesame Kale Chips	72	Coconut Almond Chia Pudding
73	Almond Butter Brownies	74	Baked Beet Chips
75	Cinnamon Roasted Nuts	76	Craneberry Coconut Trail Mix

Breakfast Recipes

Blueberry Coconut Smoothie

Servings: 1

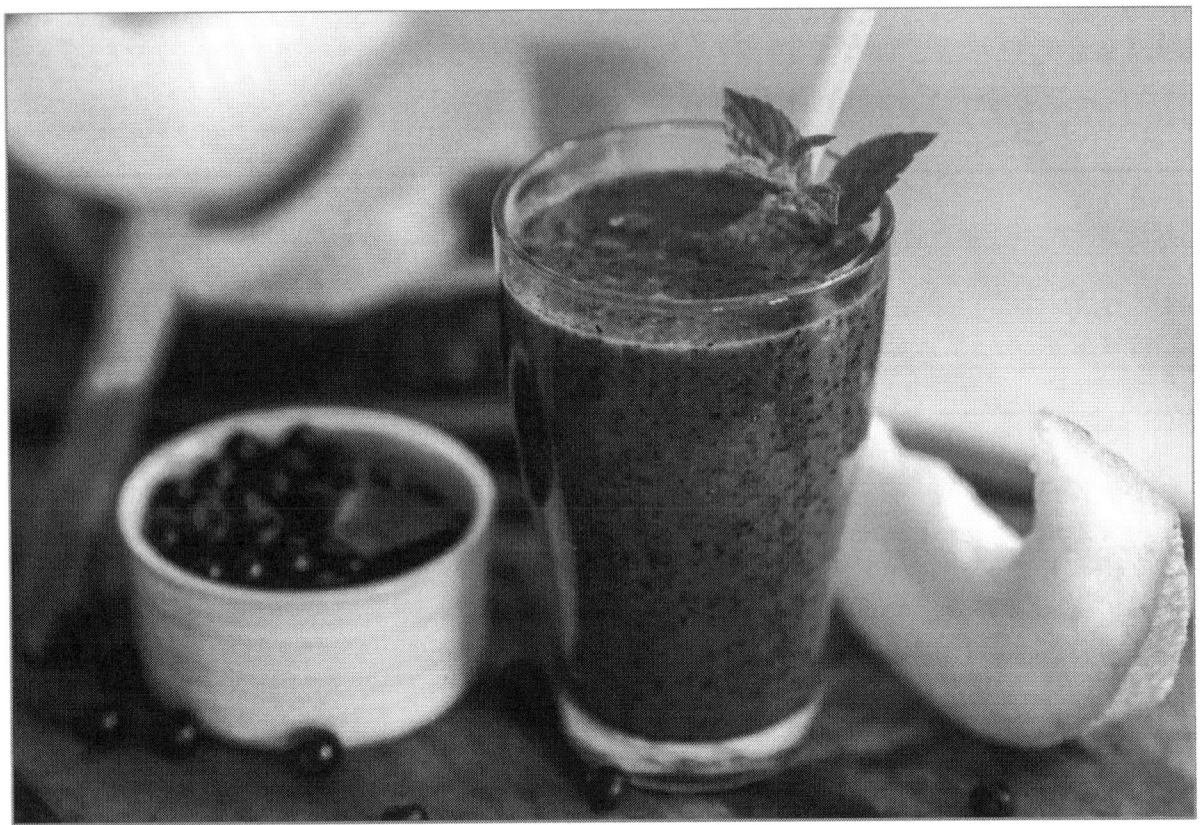

Ingredients:

- 1 cup frozen blueberries
- ½ small frozen banana, sliced
- 1 cup unsweetened coconut milk
- ¼ cup canned coconut milk
- 1 teaspoon fresh lemon juice
- Ice cubes (optional)

Instructions:

1. Combine the blueberries and coconut milk in a blender.
2. Pulse the mixture several times to chop.

3. Add the remaining ingredients.

4. Blend on high speed for 30 to 60 seconds until smooth.

5. Pour the smoothie into a glass and enjoy right away.

Tomato Basil Omelet

Servings: 1

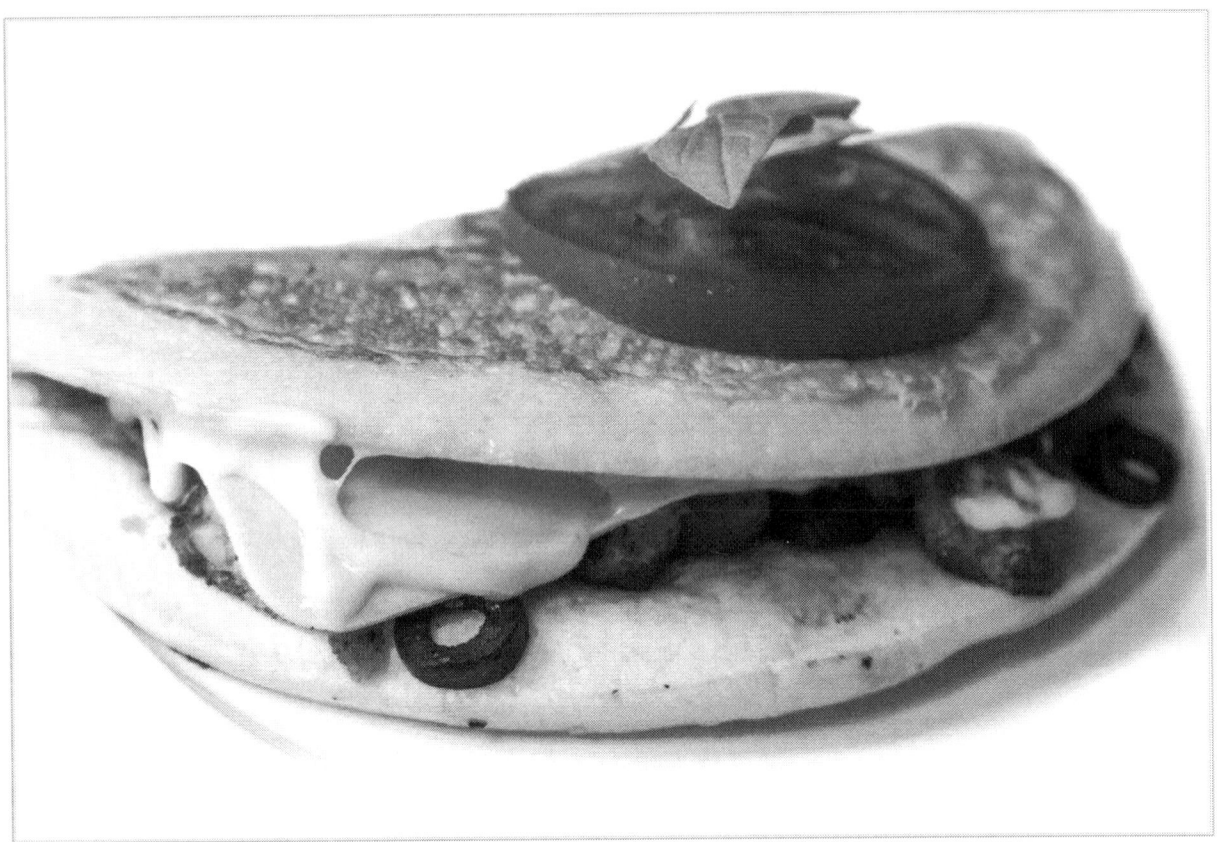

Ingredients:

- 1 teaspoon olive oil, divided
- 1 small tomato, chopped
- ¼ cup diced yellow onion
- 1 clove minced garlic
- 2 large eggs, whisked
- 1 tablespoon chopped chives
- Salt and pepper
- 1 tablespoon fresh chopped basil

Instructions:

1. Heat ½ teaspoon of olive oil in a small skillet over medium heat.
2. Add the tomato, onions, and garlic – sauté for 3 to 4 minutes until tender.
3. Spoon the vegetables off into a bowl and reheat the skillet with the remaining oil.
4. Whisk together the eggs, chives, salt and pepper.
5. Pour the egg mixture into the skillet and let it cook for 1 minute.
6. Tilt the pan to spread the uncooked egg and cook until almost set.
7. Spoon the vegetable mixture over half the omelet and sprinkle with basil.
8. Fold the omelet over and cook until the egg is set.

Spiced Apple Walnut Muffins

Servings: 1

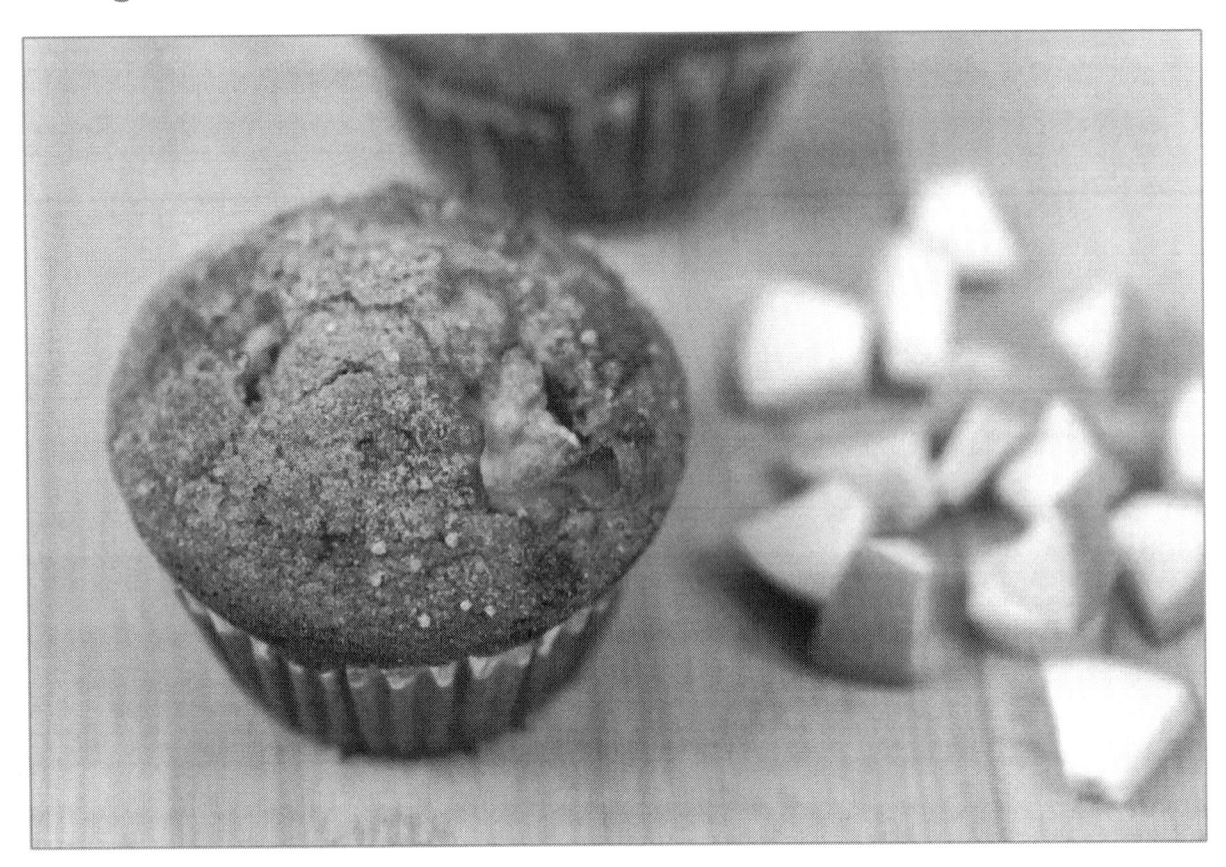

Ingredients:

- 1 ¼ cups almond flour
- 3 tablespoons coconut flour
- 2 ½ teaspoons ground cinnamon
- ½ teaspoon baking soda
- ½ teaspoon ground nutmeg
- ¼ teaspoon salt
- 2 large eggs, whisked
- 1/3 cup melted coconut oil
- ¼ cup maple syrup

- ➢ 1 tablespoon vanilla extract
- ➢ ½ cup diced apples
- ➢ ¼ cup chopped walnuts

Instructions:

1. Preheat the oven to 350°F and line 8 cups of a regular muffin pan with paper liners.
2. Combine the almond flour, coconut flour, cinnamon, baking soda, nutmeg and salt in a mixing bowl.
3. In a separate bowl, whisk together the eggs, coconut oil, maple syrup, and vanilla extract until smooth.
4. Stir the dry ingredients into the wet until just combined.
5. Fold in the chopped apples and walnuts then divide the batter evenly among the muffin cups.
6. Bake for 22 to 25 minutes until a knife inserted in the center comes out clean.
7. Cool the muffins for 5 minutes in the pan then remove to a wire cooling rack.

Ham and Red Pepper Frittata

Servings: 4

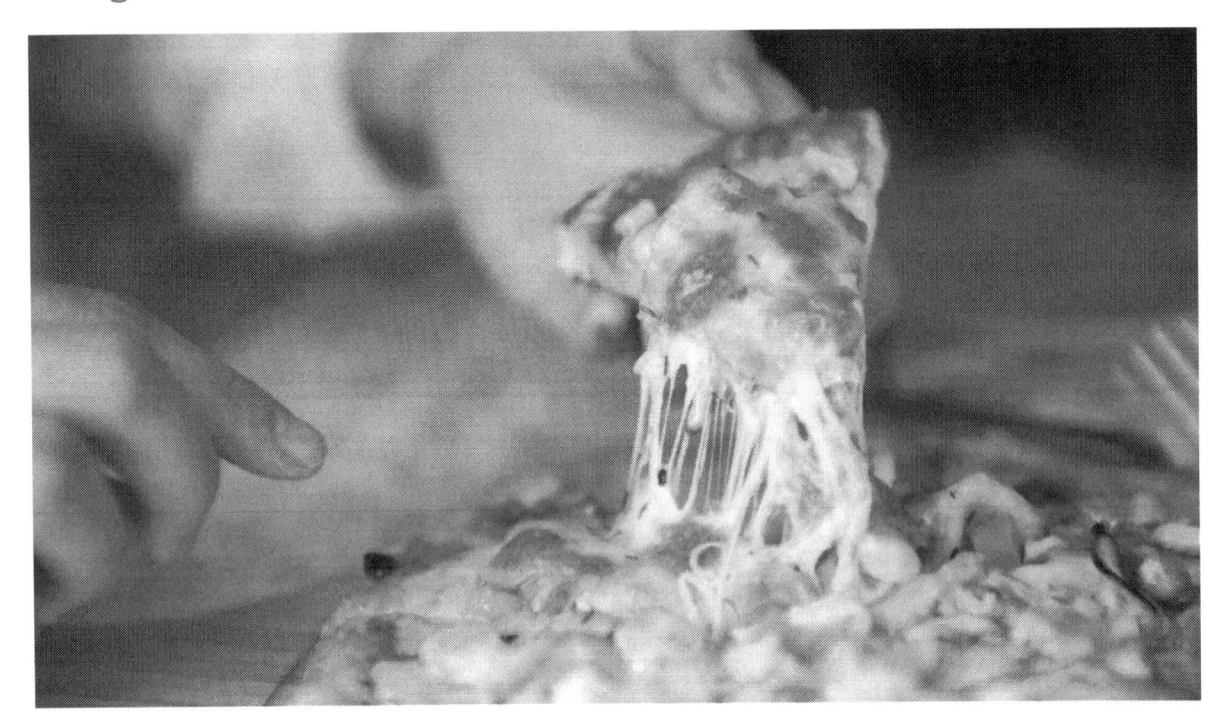

Ingredients:

- 8 large eggs, whisked
- ½ cup unsweetened almond milk
- 1 tablespoon olive oil
- 2 small red bell peppers, cored and chopped
- 1 small red onion, chopped
- 2 cloves minced garlic
- Salt and pepper
- 1 cup diced ham

Instructions:

1. Preheat the oven to 400°F.
2. Whisk together the eggs and almond milk in a bowl then set aside.

3. Heat the oil in a large oven-proof skillet over medium-high heat then add the peppers, onion, and garlic.

4. Cook for 5 to 6 minutes until the vegetables are just tender.

5. Season with salt and pepper to taste.

6. Pour the egg mixture into the skillet and sprinkle in the ham.

7. Let cook for 3 to 4 minutes until the egg begins to set around the edges.

8. Transfer the skillet to the preheated oven and cook for 10 minutes or so until the center is almost set.

9. Remove from the oven and let sit for 5 minutes before slicing to serve.

Pumpkin Pie Pancakes

Servings: 4

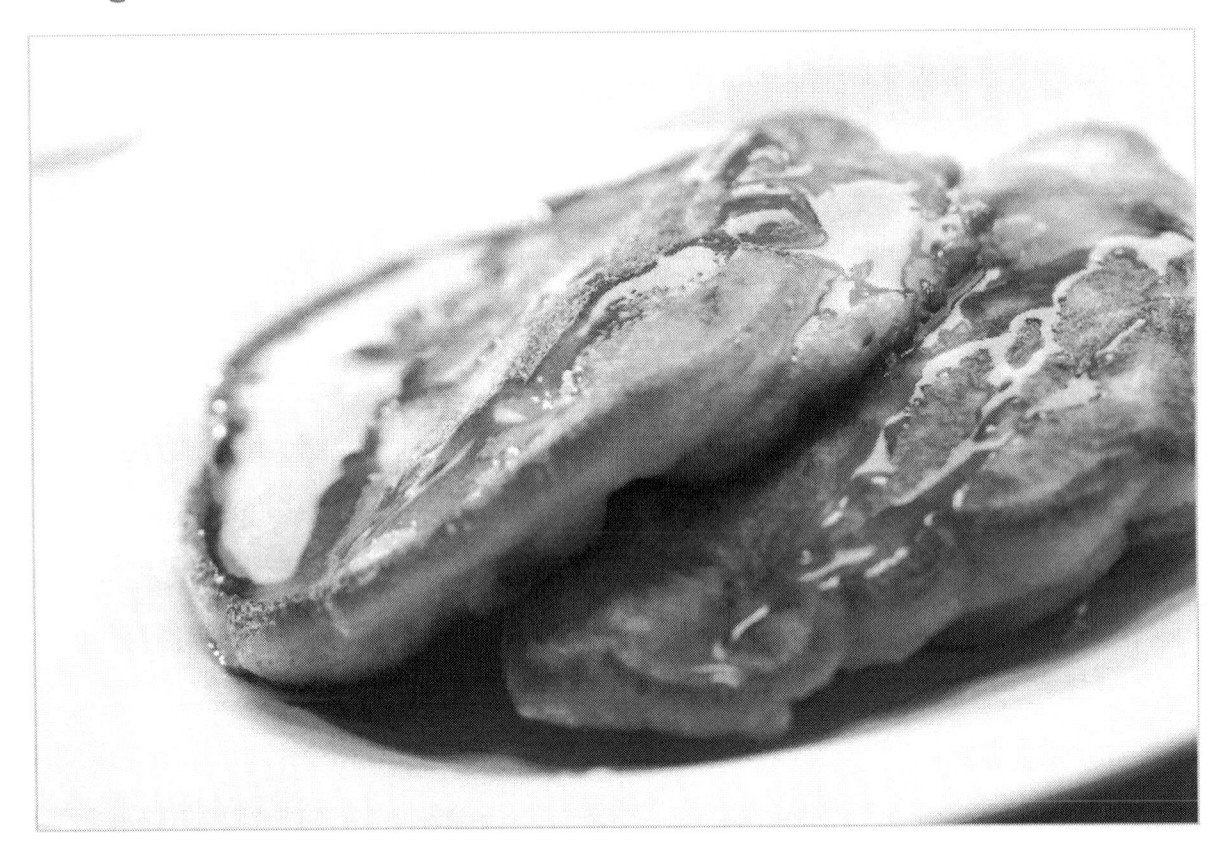

Ingredients:

- ½ cup coconut flour
- 1 cup pumpkin puree
- 4 large eggs, whisked
- ¼ cup melted coconut oil
- 2 tablespoons maple syrup
- 1 teaspoon vanilla extract
- 1 teaspoon pumpkin pie spice

Instructions:

1. Heat a large nonstick skillet over medium-high heat.

2. Combine the coconut flour, pumpkin, eggs, coconut oil, maple syrup, vanilla, and pumpkin pie spice in a food processor and blend until smooth.
3. Spoon the batter into the preheated skillet using 2 to 3 tablespoons per pancake.
4. Let the pancakes cook until bubbles begin to form on the surface.
5. Carefully flip the pancakes and let cook for 1 to 2 minutes until browned on the underside.
6. Repeat the process with the remaining batter. Serve the pancakes hot.

Strawberry Ginger Beet Smoothie

Servings: 1

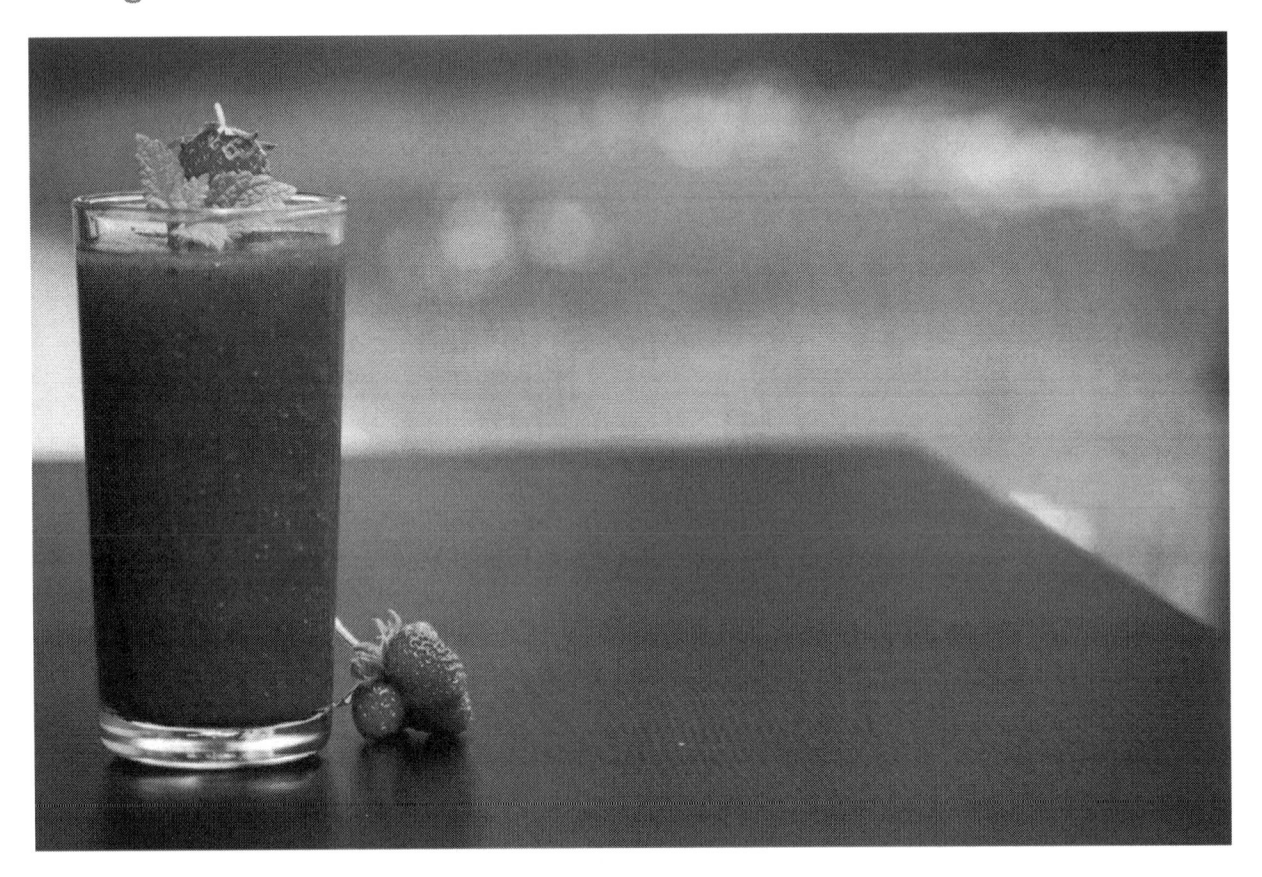

Ingredients:

- 1 ½ cups frozen sliced strawberries
- 1 small beet, peeled and chopped
- 1 cup orange juice
- ½ cup ice cubes
- 1 teaspoon fresh grated ginger

Instructions:

1. Combine the strawberries and beets in a blender.
2. Pulse the mixture several times to chop.
3. Add the remaining ingredients.

4. Blend on high speed for 30 to 60 seconds until smooth.

5. Pour the smoothie into a glass and enjoy right away.

Sweet Potato Breakfast Skillet

Servings: 4 to 5

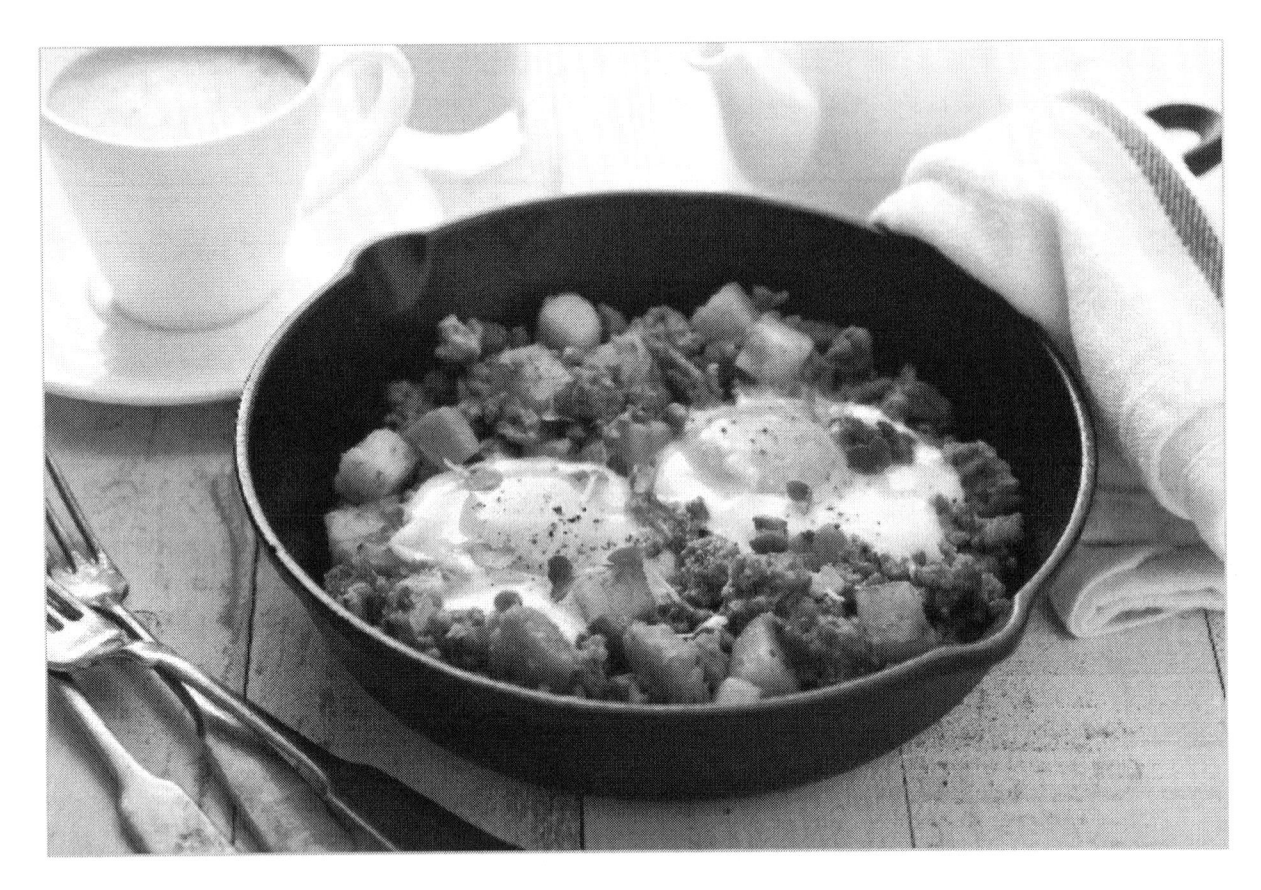

Ingredients:

- 1 pound ground sausage
- 2 large sweet potatoes, peeled and diced
- 1 medium yellow onion, diced
- 4 large eggs
- Salt and pepper
- 2 tablespoons chopped chives

Instructions:

1. Brown the sausage in an oven-proof skillet over medium-high heat.

2. Spoon the sausage into a bowl then drain the fat, reserving 1 tablespoon.

3. Heat the reserved fat over medium-high heat until hot.

4. Add the sweet potatoes and onions and sauté for 6 to 8 minutes until tender.

5. Preheat the oven to 400°F.

6. Stir the sausage back into the skillet and spread it evenly.

7. Make four depressions in the sweet potato mixture and crack an egg into each one.

8. Season with salt and pepper then place in the oven.

9. Cook for 10 to 15 minutes until the eggs are set to the desired level – sprinkle with chives to serve.

Coco-Vanilla Chia Pudding

Servings: 4

Ingredients:

- 1 (13.5-ounce) can coconut milk
- ¼ cup unsweetened almond milk
- 2 to 3 tablespoons honey
- 2 teaspoons vanilla extract
- ¼ cup chia seeds

Instructions:

1. Whisk together the coconut milk, almond milk, honey, and vanilla in a bowl.
2. Add the chia seeds and whisk until thoroughly combined.
3. Cover and chill overnight.
4. Spoon into bowls and top with fresh fruit and nuts to serve.

Spinach and Mushroom Omelet

Servings: 1

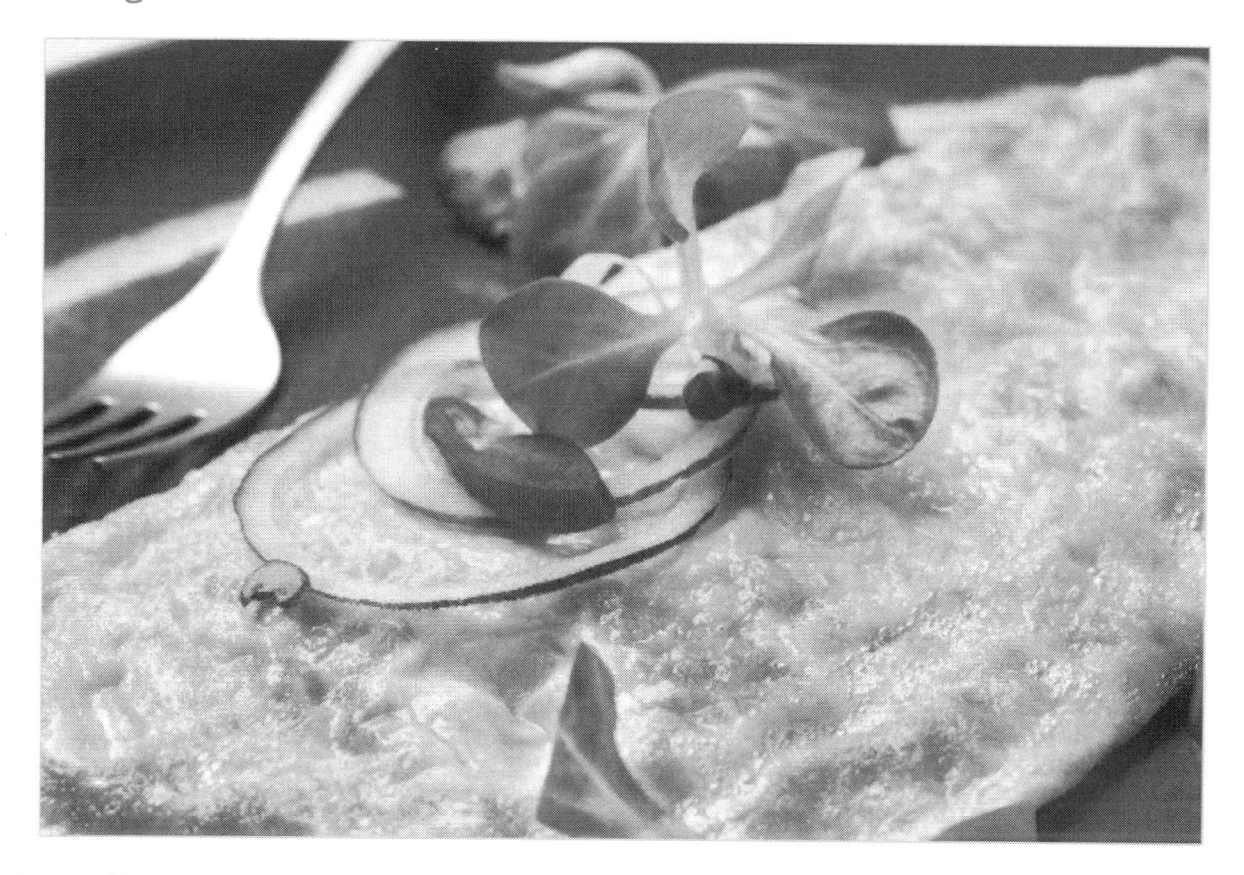

Ingredients:

- 1 teaspoon olive oil, divided
- ½ cup diced mushrooms
- ¼ cup diced yellow onion
- 1 clove minced garlic
- ¼ cup frozen spinach, thawed and drained
- 2 large eggs, whisked
- Salt and pepper

Instructions:

1. Heat ½ teaspoon of olive oil in a small skillet over medium heat.

2. Add the mushrooms, onions, and garlic – sauté for 3 to 4 minutes until tender.
3. Stir in the spinach and cook for 30 seconds or until just heated through.
4. Spoon the vegetables off into a bowl and reheat the skillet with the remaining oil.
5. Whisk together the eggs, salt and pepper.
6. Pour the egg mixture into the skillet and let it cook for 1 minute.
7. Tilt the pan to spread the uncooked egg and cook until almost set.
8. Spoon the vegetable mixture over half the omelet then fold the omelet over and cook until the egg is set.

Raspberry Kale Smoothie

Servings: 1

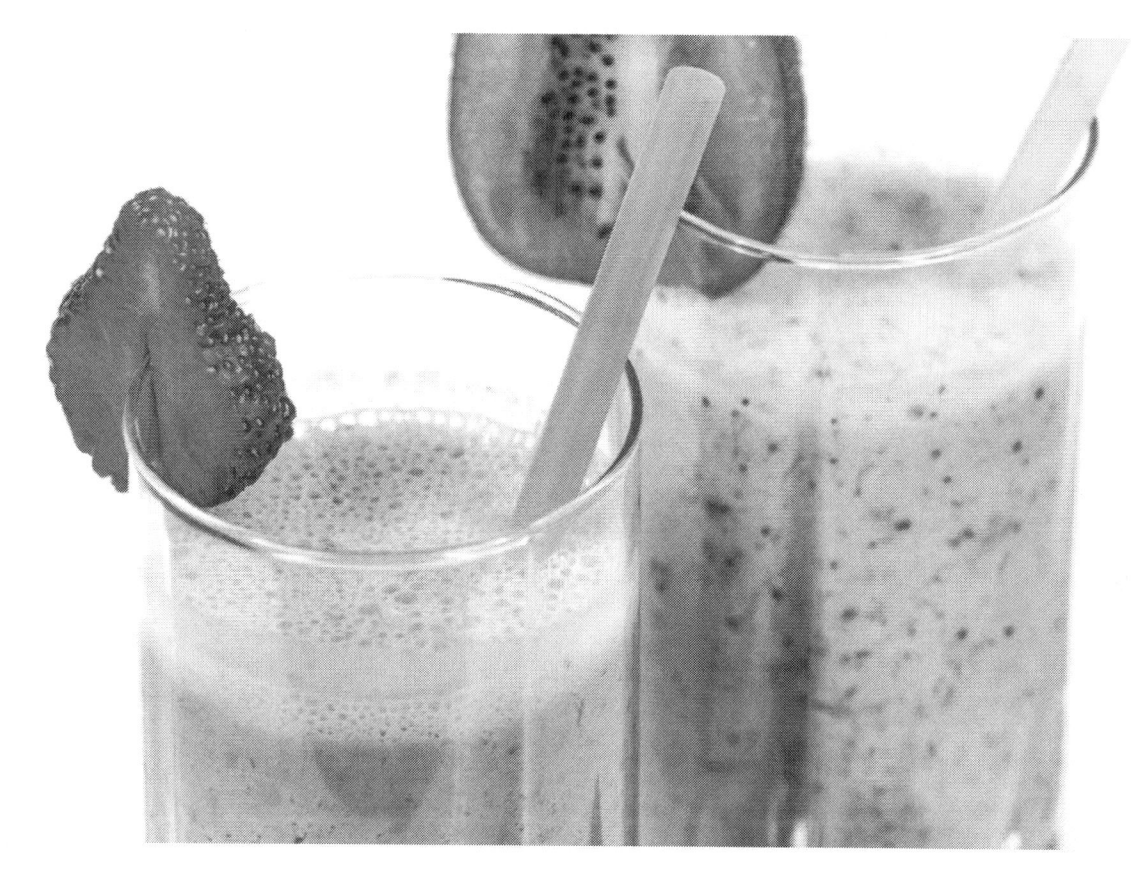

Ingredients:

- 1 cup frozen raspberries
- 1 cup fresh chopped kale
- 1 cup unsweetened apple juice
- ½ cup ice cubes
- 1 tablespoon fresh lemon juice
- 1 teaspoon honey

Instructions:

1. Combine the raspberries, kale and apple juice in a blender.
2. Pulse the mixture several times to chop.

3. Add the remaining ingredients.

4. Blend on high speed for 30 to 60 seconds until smooth.

5. Pour the smoothie into a glass and enjoy right away.

Cinnamon Banana Pancakes

Servings: 1

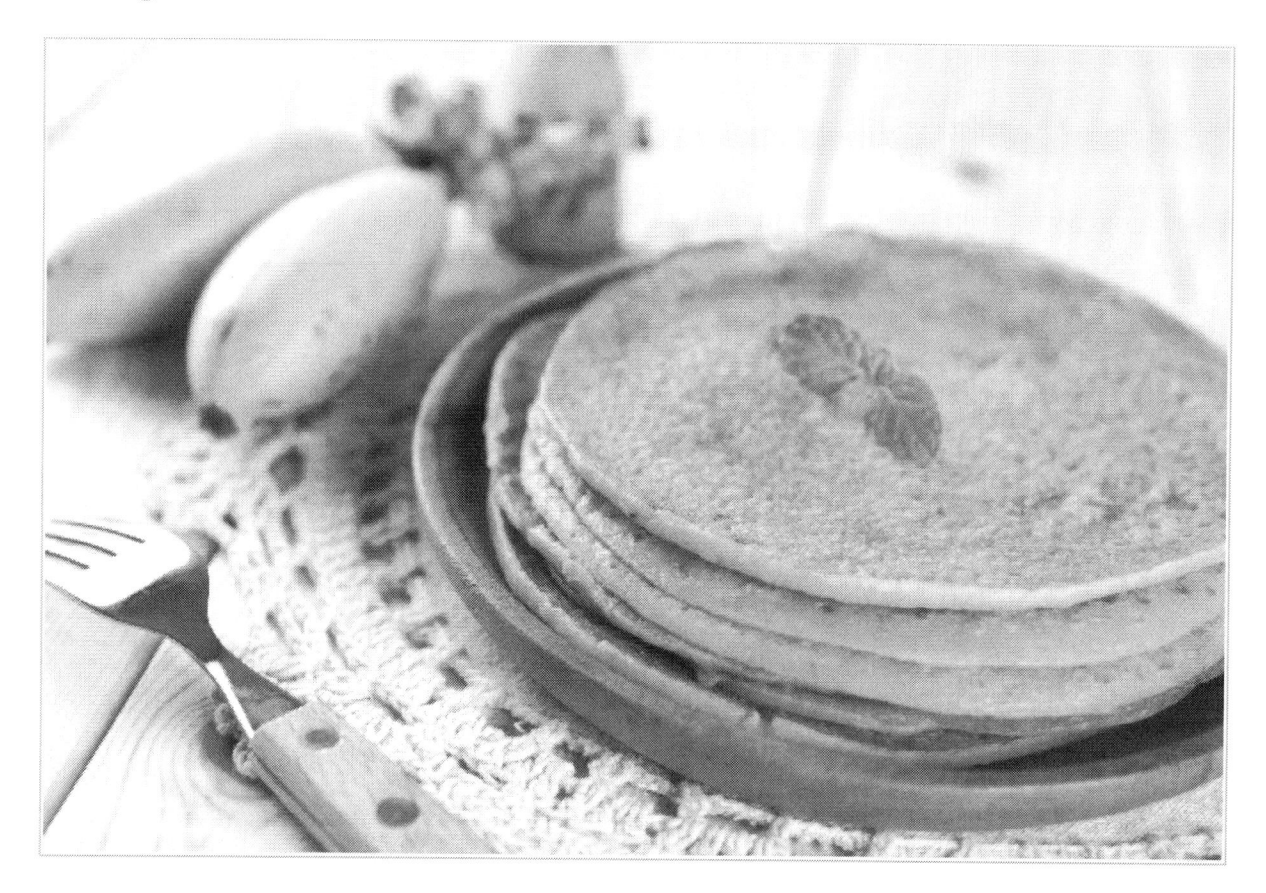

Ingredients:

- 2 large bananas, very ripe
- 2 large eggs, whisked
- ½ teaspoon vanilla extract
- ¼ teaspoon baking powder
- ¼ teaspoon ground cinnamon

Instructions:

1. Mash the bananas in a mixing bowl.
2. Stir in the eggs, baking powder, vanilla, and cinnamon.

3. Heat a large nonstick skillet over medium heat.

4. Spoon the batter into the skillet, using about 2 tablespoons per pancake.

5. Cook until the bottom is browned then carefully flip the pancakes and cook until the underside is browned.

6. Slide the pancakes onto a plate and serve with slices of fresh banana and drizzle with maple syrup.

Pumpkin Pecan Muffins

Servings: 10

Ingredients:

- 1 cup almond flour
- ½ cup coconut flour
- 2 teaspoons pumpkin pie spice
- 1 teaspoon baking soda
- ¼ teaspoon salt
- 3 large eggs, whisked
- ¾ cup pumpkin puree
- ¼ cup maple syrup
- 2 ½ tablespoons coconut oil, melted
- 1 teaspoon vanilla extract
- ¼ cup chopped pecans

Instructions:

1. Preheat the oven to 350°F and line 10 cups of a regular muffin pan with paper liners.
2. Combine the almond flour, coconut flour, pumpkin pie spice, baking soda, and salt in a mixing bowl.
3. In a separate bowl, whisk together the eggs, pumpkin, maple syrup, coconut oil, and vanilla extract until smooth.
4. Stir the dry ingredients into the wet until just combined.

5. Fold in the chopped pecans then divide the batter evenly among the muffin cups.

6. Bake for 20 to 25 minutes until a knife inserted in the center comes out clean.

7. Cool the muffins for 5 minutes in the pan then remove to a wire cooling rack.

Creamy Avocado Walnut Smoothie

Servings: 1

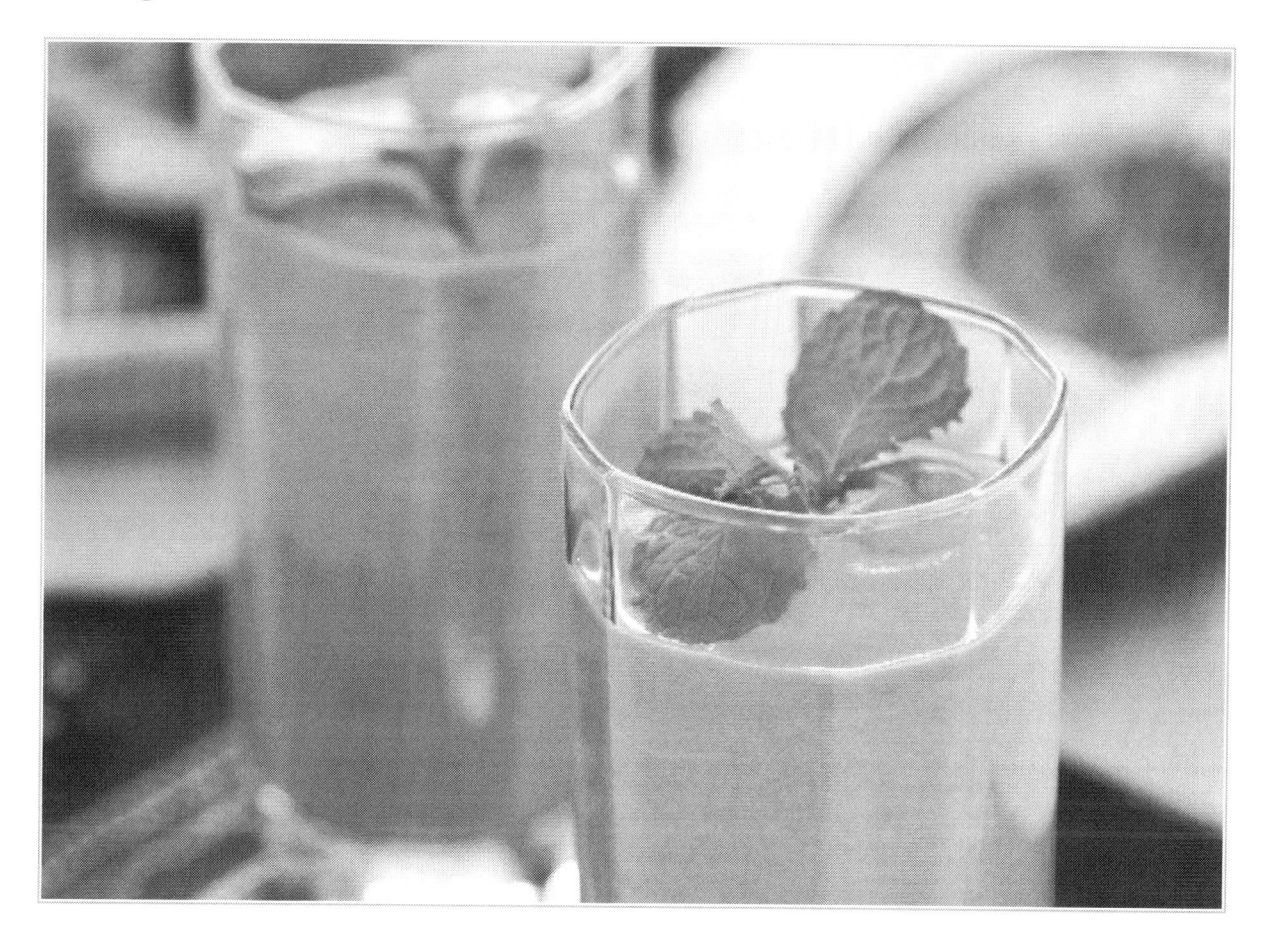

Ingredients:

- 1 large frozen banana, sliced
- ½ ripe avocado, chopped
- 1 cup unsweetened almond milk
- ½ cup ice cubes
- 2 tablespoons chopped walnuts
- Pinch ground cinnamon

Instructions:

1. Combine the banana, avocado, and almond milk in a blender.

2. Pulse the mixture several times to chop.

3. Add the remaining ingredients.

4. Blend on high speed for 30 to 60 seconds until smooth.

5. Pour the smoothie into a glass and enjoy right away.

Vegetable Egg White Omelet

Servings: 1

Ingredients:

- 1 teaspoon olive oil, divided
- 1 small tomato, chopped
- ¼ cup diced mushrooms
- ¼ cup diced yellow onion
- 2 tablespoons diced red pepper
- 1 clove minced garlic
- 3 large egg whites, whisked
- 1 tablespoon chopped chives
- Salt and pepper

Instructions:

1. Heat ½ teaspoon of olive oil in a small skillet over medium heat.
2. Add the vegetables and garlic – sauté for 3 to 4 minutes until tender.
3. Spoon the vegetables off into a bowl and reheat the skillet with the remaining oil.
4. Whisk together the eggs, chives, salt and pepper.
5. Pour the egg mixture into the skillet and let it cook for 1 minute.
6. Tilt the pan to spread the uncooked egg and cook until almost set.
7. Spoon the vegetable mixture over half the omelet.
8. Fold the omelet over and cook until the egg is set.

Cinnamon Coconut Flour Waffles

Servings: 4

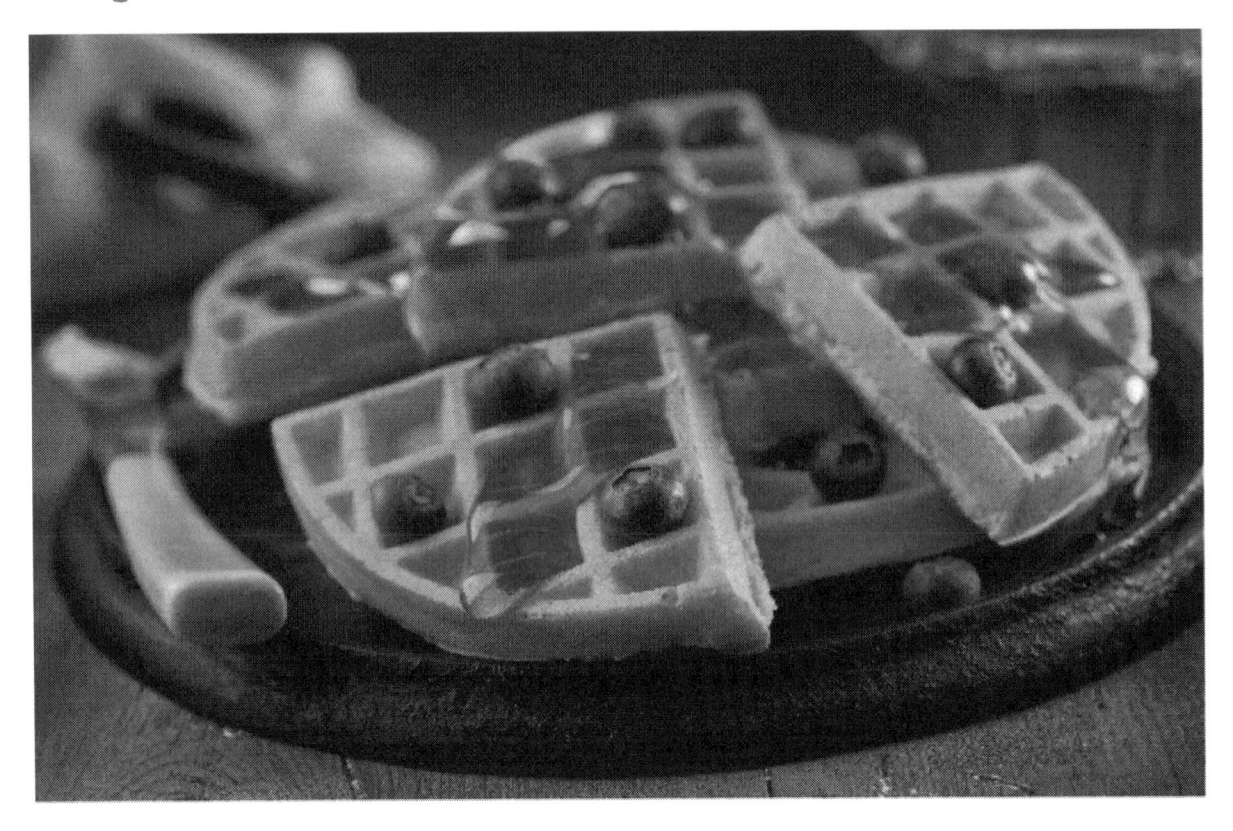

Ingredients:

- 8 large eggs, whisked well
- ½ cup coconut oil, melted
- 1 ½ teaspoons vanilla extract
- ½ teaspoon ground cinnamon
- ¼ teaspoon salt
- ½ cup coconut flour

Instructions:

1. Preheat a waffle iron and grease lightly with cooking spray.

2. Whisk the eggs in a medium mixing bowl with the coconut oil, vanilla extract, cinnamon and salt.
3. Add the coconut flour in small batches, whisking smooth after each addition.
4. Spoon ¼ cup of the batter into the preheated waffle iron and close the lid.
5. Cook the waffle for 2 to 4 minutes until lightly browned.
6. Carefully remove the waffle to a plate and repeat the procedure with the remaining waffles.
7. Serve drizzled with pure maple syrup.

Triple Berry Smoothie

Servings: 1

Ingredients:

- 1 cup frozen sliced strawberries
- ½ cup frozen raspberries
- ½ cup frozen blueberries
- 1 cup unsweetened almond milk
- ¼ cup canned coconut milk
- 1 teaspoon fresh lemon juice

Instructions:

1. Combine the berries and almond milk in a blender.
2. Pulse the mixture several times to chop.
3. Add the remaining ingredients.
4. Blend on high speed for 30 to 60 seconds until smooth.
5. Pour the smoothie into a glass and enjoy right away.

Mixed Vegetable Frittata

Servings: 4

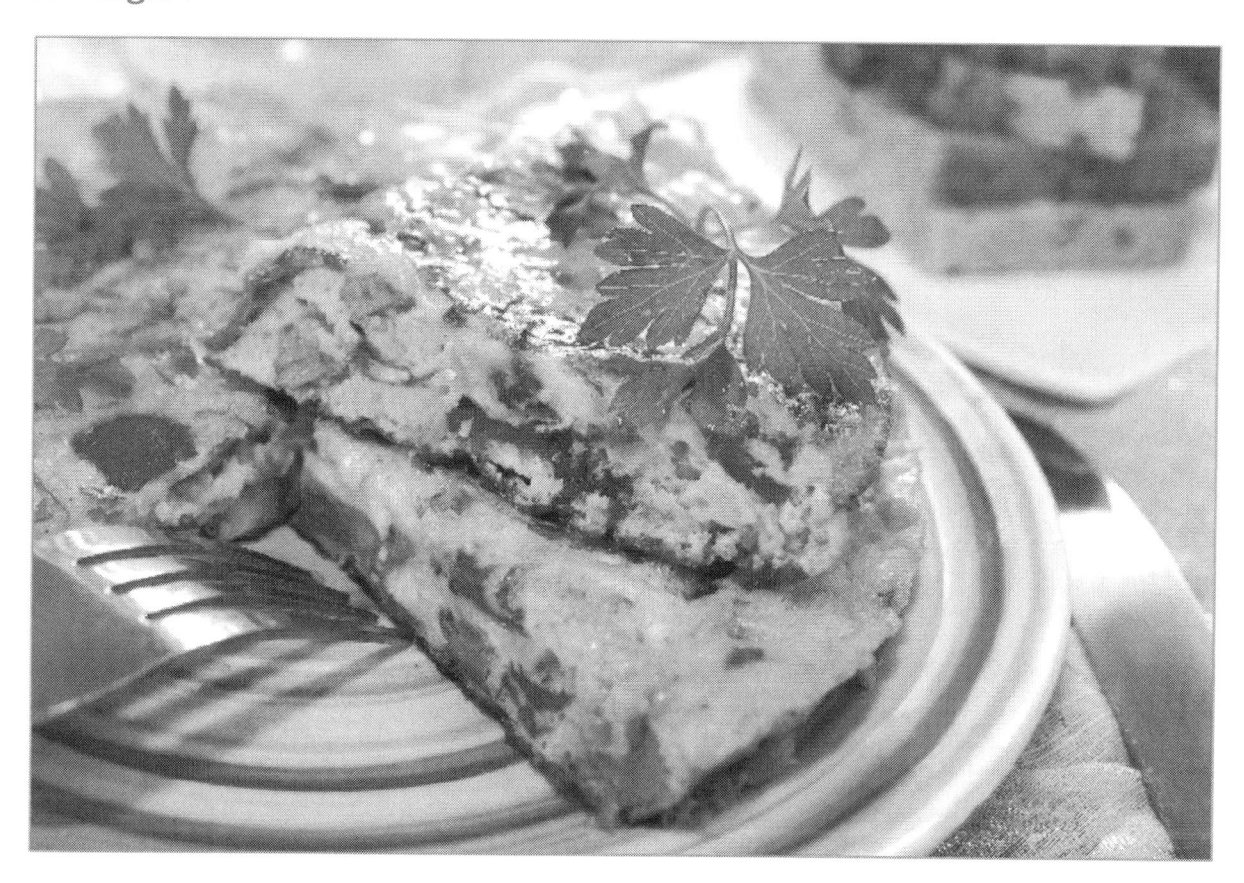

Ingredients:

- 8 large eggs, whisked
- ½ cup unsweetened almond milk
- 1 tablespoon olive oil
- 1 medium onion, chopped
- 1 small bell pepper, cored and chopped
- ½ cup diced broccoli florets
- ½ cup diced tomatoes
- 2 cloves minced garlic
- Salt and pepper

Instructions:

1. Preheat the oven to 400°F.
2. Whisk together the eggs and almond milk in a bowl then set aside.
3. Heat the oil in a large oven-proof skillet over medium-high heat.
4. Add the onion, peppers, broccoli, tomato, and garlic.
5. Cook for 5 to 6 minutes until the vegetables are just tender.
6. Season with salt and pepper to taste.
7. Pour the egg mixture into the skillet and let cook for 3 to 4 minutes until the egg begins to set around the edges.
8. Transfer the skillet to the preheated oven and cook for 10 minutes or so until the center is almost set.
9. Remove from the oven and let sit for 5 minutes before slicing to serve.

Sweet Apple Pancakes

Servings: 4

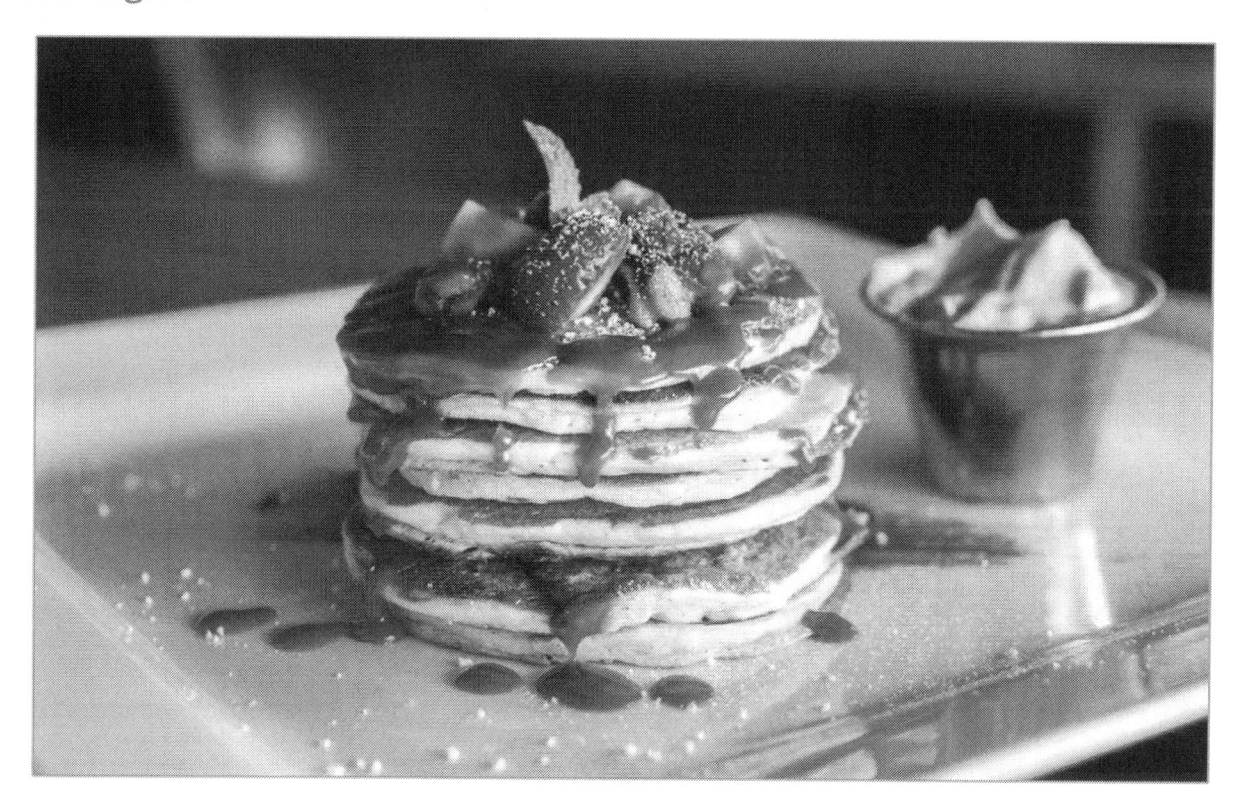

Ingredients:

- ½ cup coconut flour
- 1 cup unsweetened applesauce
- 4 large eggs, whisked
- ¼ cup melted coconut oil
- 2 tablespoons honey
- 1 teaspoon vanilla extract
- 1 to 2 cups diced apples

Instructions:

1. Heat a large nonstick skillet over medium-high heat.

2. Combine the coconut flour, applesauce, eggs, coconut oil, honey, and vanilla in a food processor and blend until smooth.
3. Spoon the batter into the preheated skillet using 2 to 3 tablespoons per pancake.
4. Sprinkle a handful of chopped apples into the wet batter of each pancake.
5. Let the pancakes cook until bubbles begin to form on the surface.
6. Carefully flip the pancakes and let cook for 1 to 2 minutes until browned on the underside.
7. Repeat the process with the remaining batter. Serve the pancakes hot.

Blueberry Muffins

Servings: 8

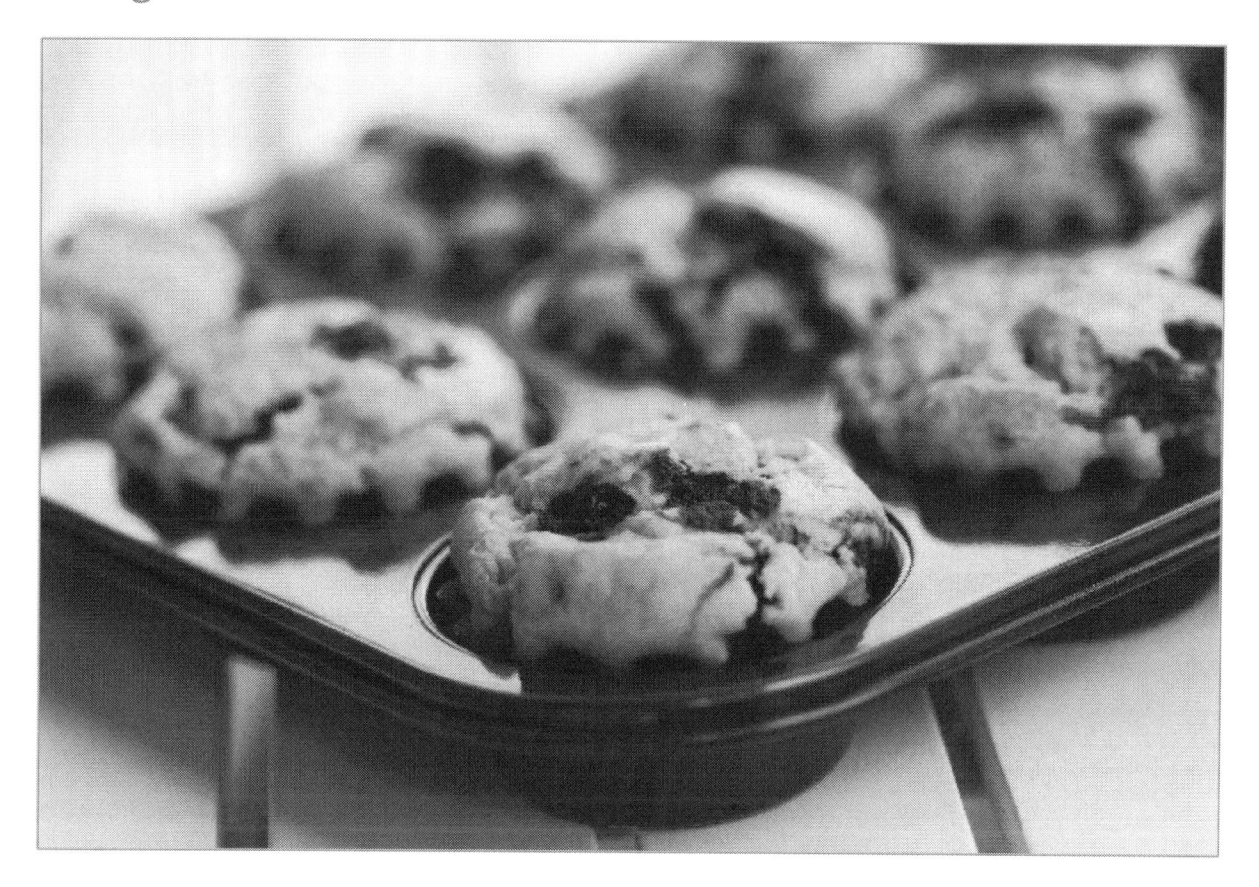

Ingredients:

- 1 ¼ cups almond flour
- 3 tablespoons coconut flour
- ½ teaspoon baking soda
- ¼ teaspoon salt
- 2 large eggs, whisked
- 1/3 cup melted coconut oil
- ¼ cup honey
- 1 teaspoon vanilla extract
- 1 cup fresh blueberries

Instructions:

1. Preheat the oven to 350°F and line 8 cups of a regular muffin pan with paper liners.
2. Combine the almond flour, coconut flour, baking soda, and salt in a mixing bowl.
3. In a separate bowl, whisk together the eggs, coconut oil, honey, and vanilla extract until smooth.
4. Stir the dry ingredients into the wet until just combined.
5. Fold in the blueberries then divide the batter evenly among the muffin cups.
6. Bake for 22 to 25 minutes until a knife inserted in the center comes out clean.
7. Cool the muffins for 5 minutes in the pan then remove to a wire cooling rack.

Almond Butter Banana Smoothie

Servings: 1

Ingredients:

- 1 large frozen banana, sliced
- 1 cup unsweetened almond milk
- ½ cup ice cubes
- 2 tablespoons almond butter
- Pinch ground cinnamon

Instructions:

1. Combine the banana and almond milk in a blender.
2. Pulse the mixture several times to chop.
3. Add the remaining ingredients.
4. Blend on high speed for 30 to 60 seconds until smooth.
5. Pour the smoothie into a glass and enjoy right away.

Lunch Recipes

Curried Butternut Squash Soup

Servings: 4 to 6

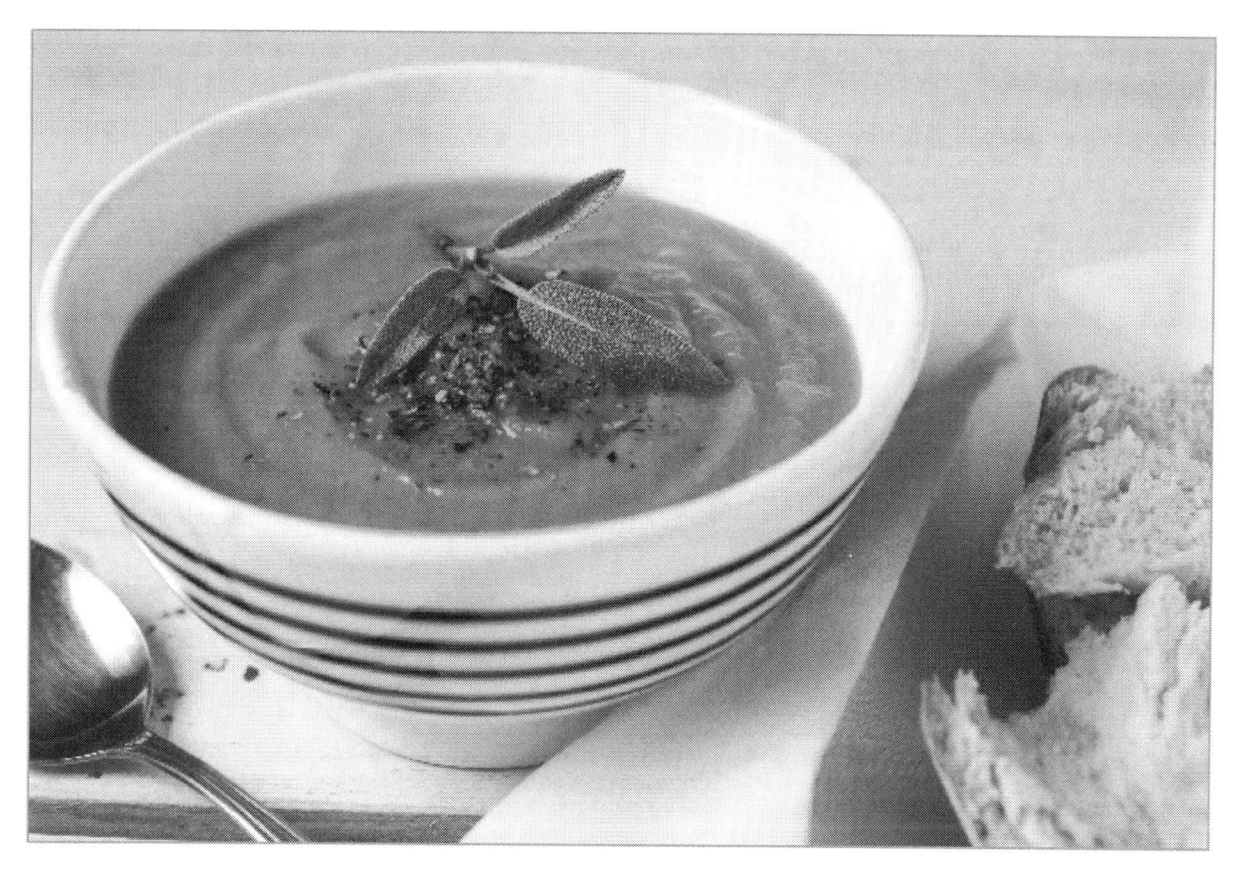

Ingredients:

- 2 tablespoons olive oil, divided
- 6 cups chopped butternut squash
- 1 large sweet onion, chopped
- 1 tablespoon fresh grated ginger
- 1 tablespoon minced garlic
- 2 teaspoons curry powder
- ¼ teaspoon ground mustard powder
- Salt and pepper to taste
- 4 cups chicken stock (low sodium)

Instructions:

1. Heat 1 tablespoon oil in a large saucepan over medium heat.
2. Add the butternut squash and sauté for 6 to 8 minutes until browned.
3. Spoon the squash into a bowl and reheat the skillet with the remaining oil.
4. Add the onions, curry powder, garlic, ginger, mustard powder, salt and pepper.
5. Cook for 4 to 6 minutes until the onions are translucent.
6. Add the squash back to the pot along with the chicken stock.
7. Bring to a boil then reduce heat and simmer, covered, for 45 minutes.
8. Turn off the heat and puree the soup using an immersion blender until smooth.
9. Spoon into bowls and serve hot.

Avocado Egg Salad

Servings: 4

Ingredients:

- 6 large hardboiled eggs, peeled and chopped
- 1 large ripe avocado, pitted and diced
- 2 tablespoons fresh lemon juice
- 6 slices cooked bacon, crumbled
- 2 green onions, sliced thin
- Paprika to taste

Instructions:

1. Combine the avocado and hardboiled egg in a bowl.
2. Mash the two ingredients together using a fork.
3. Stir in the lemon juice and salt then toss in the bacon and green onion.
4. Season with paprika to taste then chill until ready to serve.

Roasted Tomato Basil Soup

Servings: 4 to 6

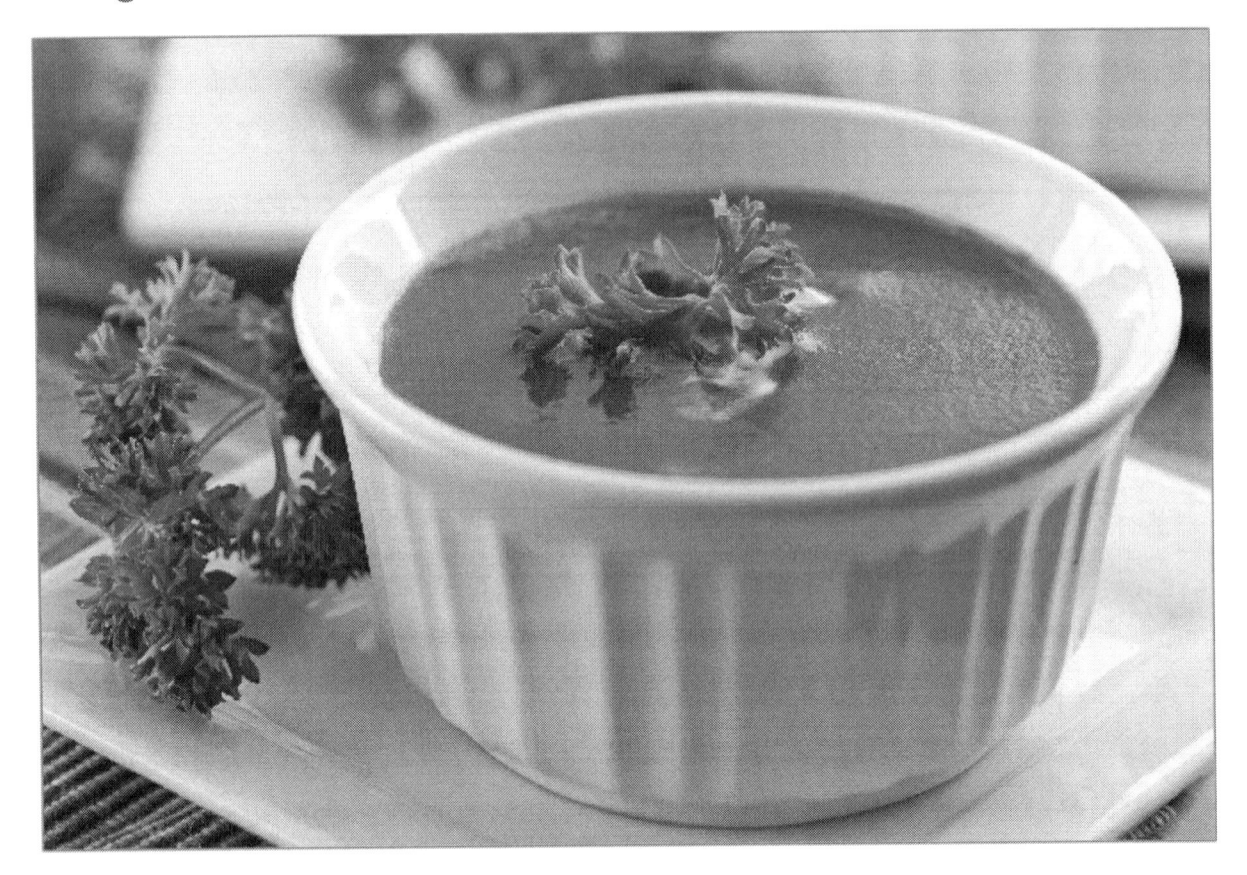

Ingredients:

- 4 large vine-ripened tomatoes, sliced
- 1 large sweet onion, sliced
- 6 cloves fresh garlic, sliced
- Olive oil, as needed
- Salt and pepper
- 2 cups vegetable broth
- 2 tablespoons tomato paste
- ¼ cup fresh chopped basil

Instructions:

1. Preheat the oven to 350°F.
2. Spread the tomatoes, onions, and garlic on a foil-lined baking sheet and drizzle with oil.
3. Season with salt and pepper then toss gently.
4. Roast for 40 minutes, stirring once halfway through, until very tender.
5. Heat the vegetable stock in a large saucepan over medium heat.
6. Whisk in the tomato paste and basil then add the roasted vegetables.
7. Bring to a boil then reduce heat and simmer, covered, for 10 minutes.
8. Turn off the heat and puree the soup using an immersion blender until smooth.
9. Spoon into bowls and serve hot.

Avocado Spinach Salad with Egg

Servings: 4

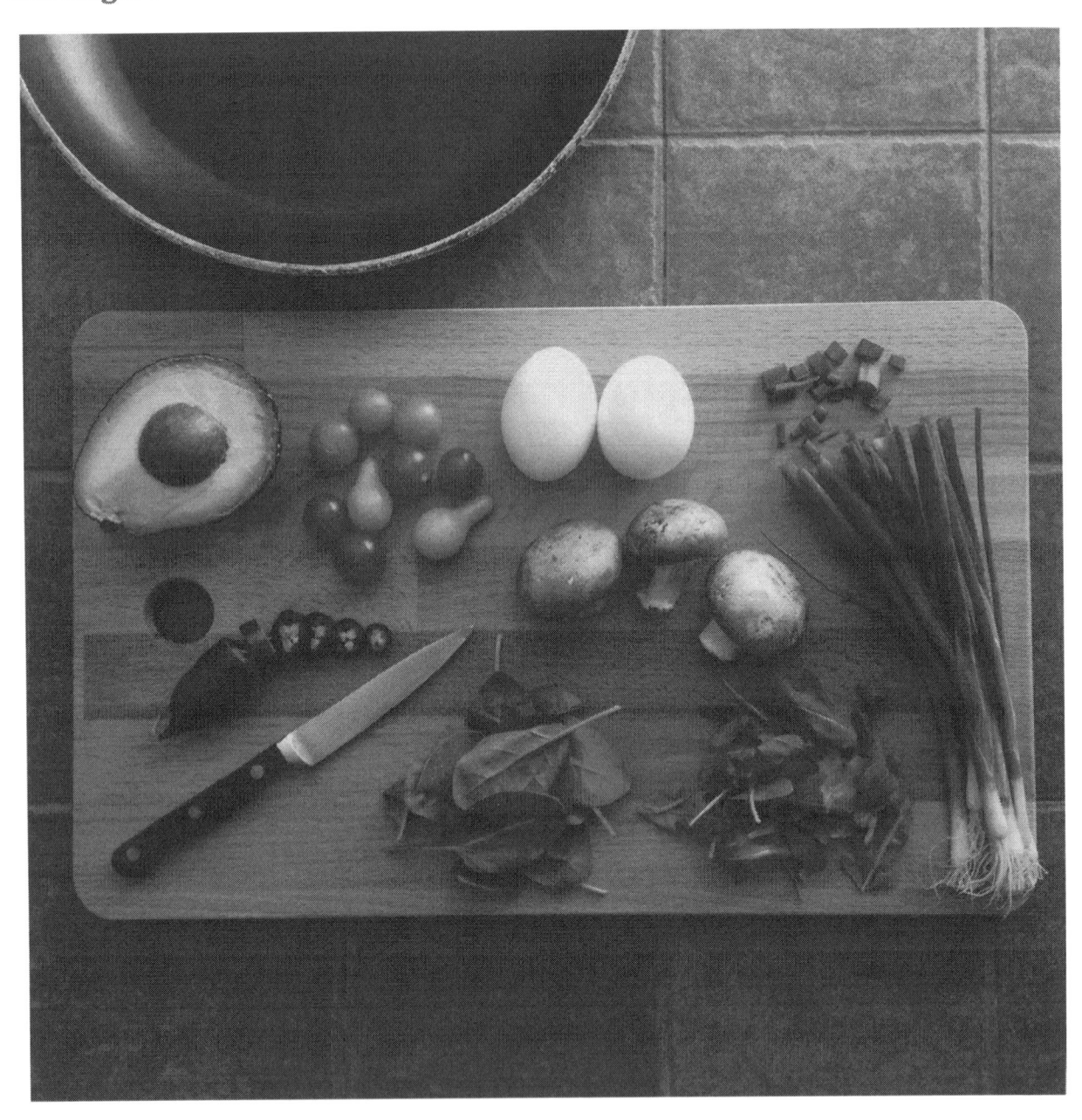

Ingredients:

- 5 cups fresh baby spinach
- 1 cup thinly sliced mushrooms
- ½ small red onion, sliced thin

- 1 large avocado, pitted and sliced thin
- 4 hardboiled eggs, peeled and sliced

Instructions:

1. Combine the spinach, mushrooms, and red onion in a large salad bowl.
2. Toss well then divide among four salad plates.
3. Top each salad with slices of avocado and hardboiled egg.
4. Drizzle with your favorite paleo dressing to serve.

Creamy Sweet Potato Soup

Servings: 4

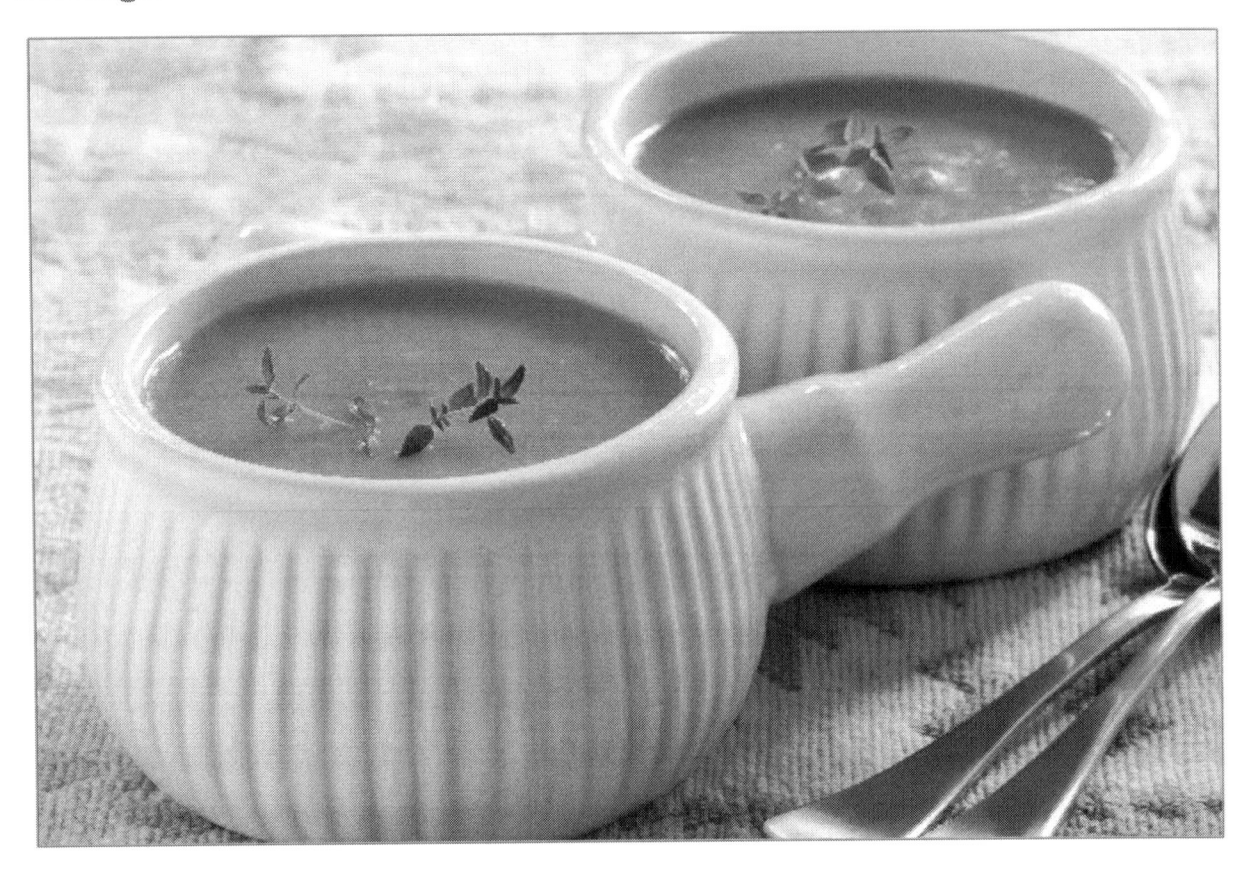

Ingredients:

- 1 tablespoon coconut oil
- 2 medium sweet onions, chopped
- 3 cloves minced garlic
- 6 cups chopped sweet potatoes
- 4 cups chicken broth (low sodium)
- ½ teaspoon ground cinnamon
- Salt and pepper

Instructions:

1. Heat the coconut oil in a large saucepan over medium-high heat.

2. Stir in the onions and garlic then cook for 5 to 6 minutes until tender.

3. Add the sweet potatoes and sauté for 5 minutes.

4. Stir in the broth then bring to a boil.

5. Reduce heat and simmer, covered, for 20 minutes until the vegetables are tender.

6. Turn off the heat and puree the soup using an immersion blender until smooth.

7. Season with cinnamon, salt and pepper and serve hot.

Apple Walnut Chicken Salad

Servings: 4

Ingredients:

- 2 tablespoons olive oil
- 1 tablespoon fresh lemon juice
- 2 tablespoons fresh chopped parsley
- 2 cloves minced garlic
- Salt and pepper to taste
- 2 cups cooked chicken breast, chopped
- 1 small ripe avocado, pitted and chopped
- 1 small green apple, peeled and diced
- ¼ cup diced celery
- ¼ cup sliced green onion
- ¼ cup chopped walnuts

Instructions:

1. Whisk together the olive oil, lemon juice, parsley, garlic, salt and pepper in a mixing bowl.
2. Toss in the cooked chicken, avocado, apple, celery, green onion, and walnuts until evenly coated.
3. Serve on a bed of lettuce.

Hearty Beef and Vegetable Stew

Servings: 4

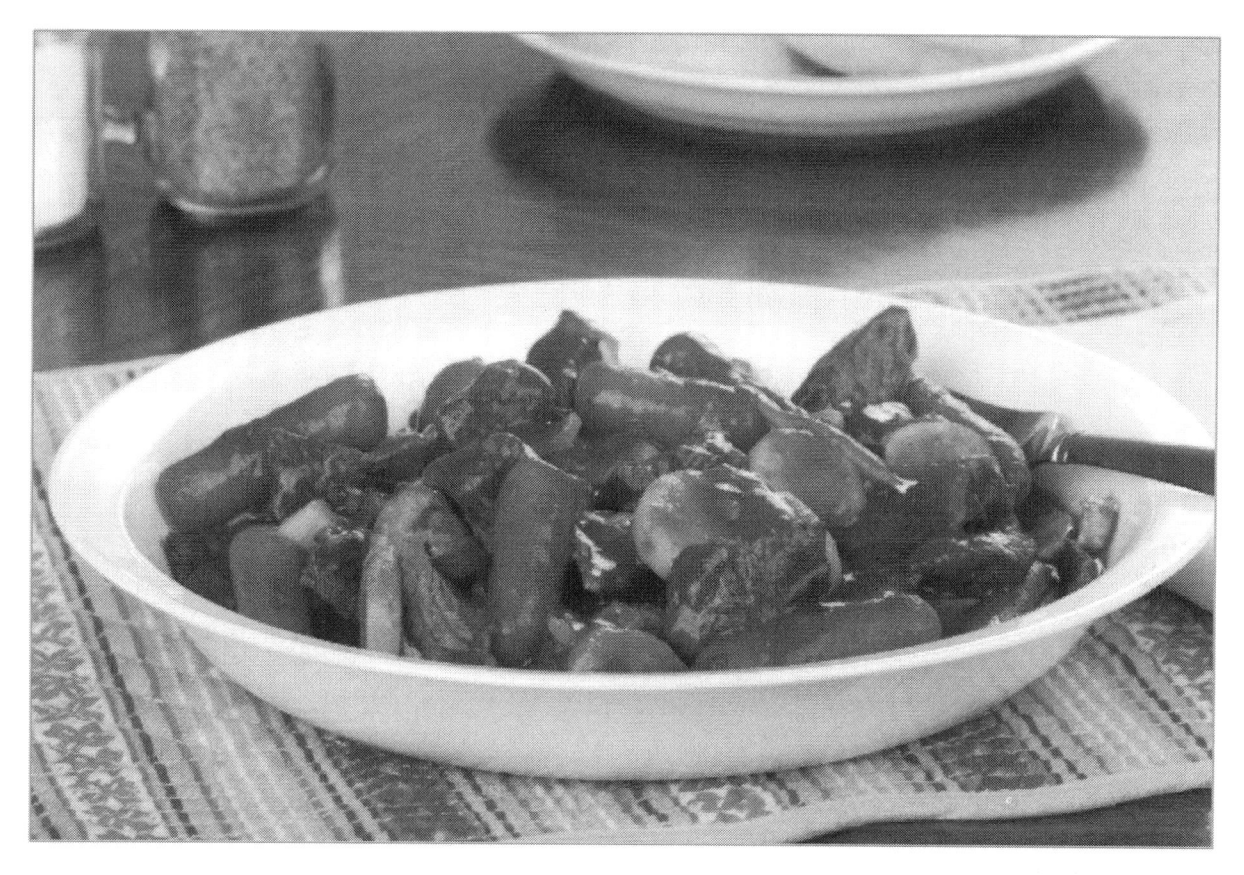

Ingredients:

- 1 tablespoon olive oil
- 2 medium sweet potatoes, peeled and chopped
- 2 large carrots, peeled and sliced
- 1 large yellow onion, chopped
- 1 cup sliced celery
- 1 pound beef stew meat, chopped
- 2 (14-ounce) cans diced tomatoes
- 4 cups beef stock (low sodium)
- 1 teaspoon fresh chopped rosemary

- ➢ ½ teaspoon fresh chopped thyme
- ➢ Salt and pepper

Instructions:

1. Heat the oil in a large saucepan over medium-high heat.
2. Add the sweet potatoes, carrots, onion, and celery and cook for 4 to 5 minutes until lightly browned.
3. Stir in the beef along with the tomatoes, stock, and seasonings.
4. Bring the mixture to a boil then reduce heat and simmer, covered, for one hour – stir every 15 minutes.
5. Uncover the pot and simmer for another 45 minutes then serve hot.

Balsamic Strawberry Kale Salad

Servings: 4

Ingredients:

- 6 tablespoons olive oil
- 2 tablespoons balsamic vinegar
- 2 teaspoons Dijon mustard
- 1 clove minced garlic
- Pinch salt and pepper
- 5 to 6 cups fresh chopped kale
- 1 ½ cups sliced strawberries
- ½ small red onion, sliced thin

Instructions:

1. Combine the olive oil, balsamic vinegar, mustard, garlic, salt and pepper in a bowl and whisk until thoroughly combined.
2. Add the kale, strawberries, and red onion.
3. Toss until evenly coated then divide among salad plates to serve.

Cream of Broccoli Soup

Servings: 4 to 5

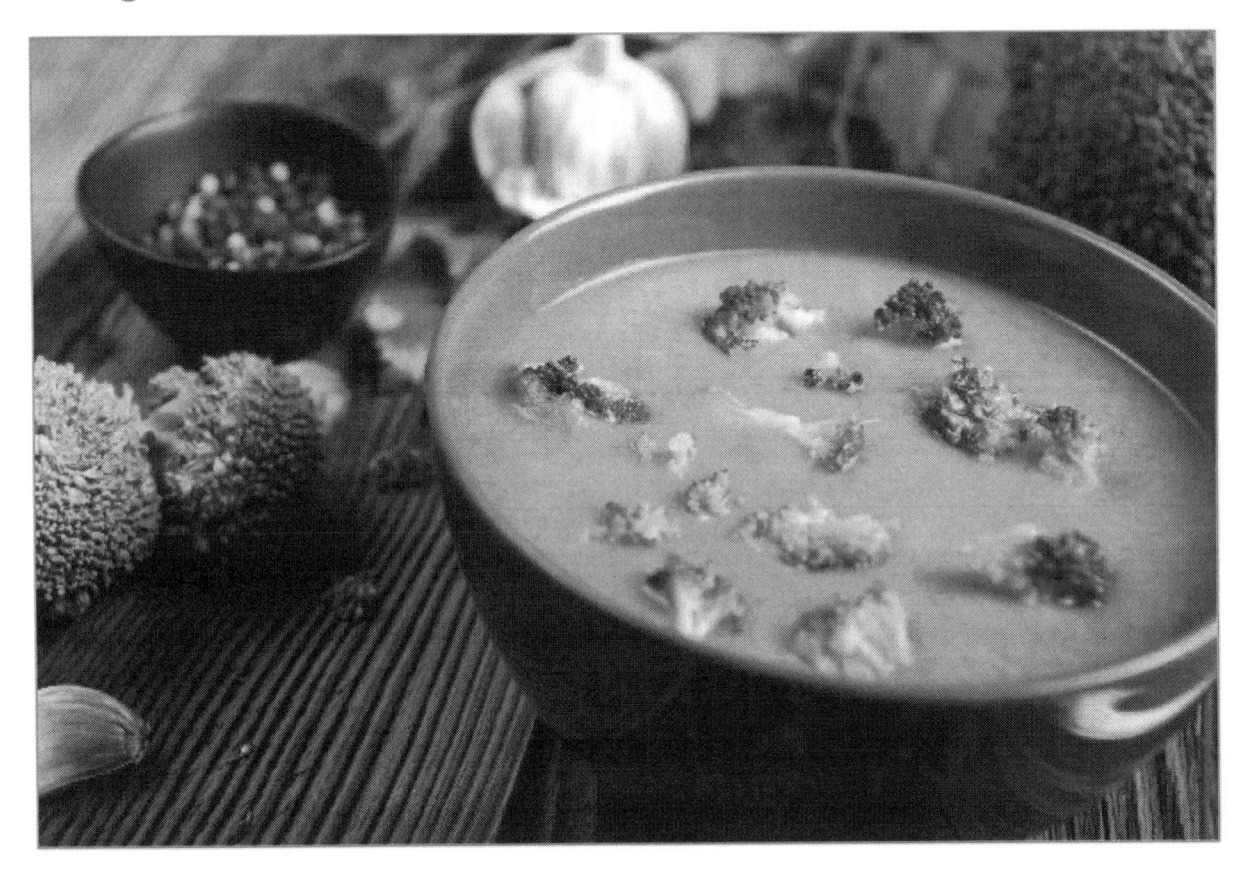

Ingredients:

- 1 tablespoon olive oil
- 1 medium white onion, chopped
- 2 cloves minced garlic
- 3 cups chicken broth (low sodium)
- 1 pound fresh chopped broccoli
- 1 medium leek, sliced (white and light green parts only)
- Salt and pepper
- 1 cup canned coconut milk

Instructions:

1. Heat the oil in a large saucepan over medium-high heat.
2. Add the onions and cook for 4 to 5 minutes until translucent.
3. Stir in the garlic and cook for 1 minute more.
4. Add the broth, broccoli, and leeks then season with salt and pepper.
5. Bring to a boil then reduce heat and simmer for 20 minutes until the broccoli is very tender.
6. Turn off the heat and puree the soup using an immersion blender.
7. Stir in the coconut milk and adjust seasoning to taste. Serve hot.

Chopped Chicken and Mango Salad

Servings: 4

Ingredients:

- 1 tablespoon olive oil
- 1 pound boneless skinless chicken breast, chopped
- 1 teaspoon chili powder
- Salt and pepper
- ½ cup olive oil mayonnaise
- 1 ½ tablespoons fresh lime juice
- 3 cloves minced garlic
- ½ red pepper, cored and diced
- ¼ cup diced red onion
- 1 ripe mango, peeled and diced

Instructions:

1. Heat the oil in a large skillet over medium-high heat.
2. Add the chicken and season with chili powder, salt and pepper.
3. Sauté the chicken until evenly browned and cooked through then remove to a bowl and let cool.
4. Combine the mayonnaise, lime juice, and garlic in a mixing bowl.
5. Whisk well then toss in the chopped chicken, bell pepper, red onion, and mango.
6. Chill until ready to serve then serve over a bed of lettuce.

Mushroom and Leek Soup

Servings: 4 to 6

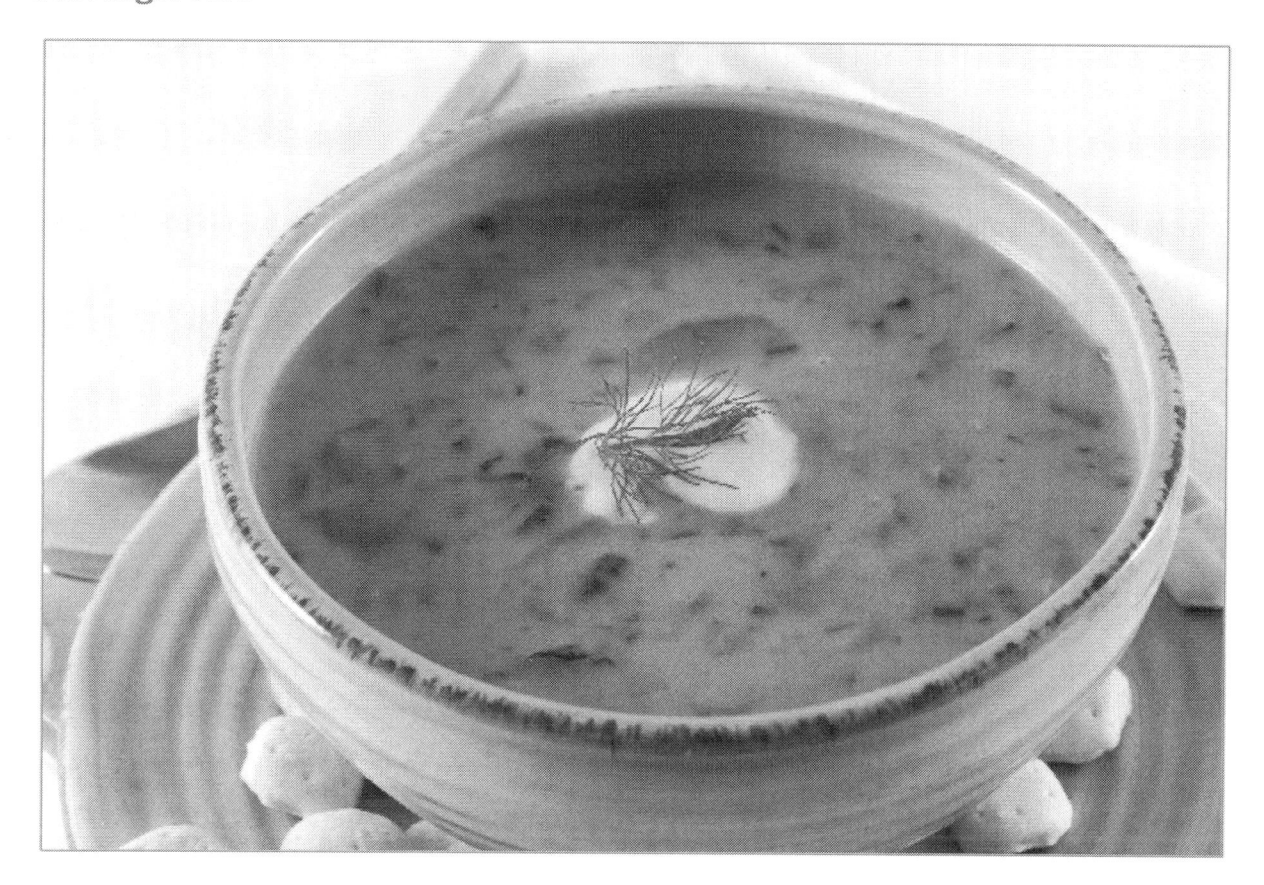

Ingredients:

- 1 tablespoon olive oil
- 1 large leek, sliced thin (white and light green parts only)
- 1 ½ pounds fresh sliced mushrooms
- 1 small white onion, chopped
- 3 cloves minced garlic
- 2 cups vegetable broth (divided)
- 2 tablespoons arrowroot powder
- ¼ cup canned coconut milk
- 1 tablespoon fresh chopped thyme

- ➢ 1 tablespoon fresh chopped rosemary
- ➢ Salt and pepper, to taste

Instructions:

1. Heat the oil in a large saucepan over medium heat.
2. Add the leeks and cook for 4 to 5 minutes until just browned.
3. Stir in the mushrooms, onion, and garlic and cook for 6 to 8 minutes until tender.
4. Pour in 2 tablespoons of the vegetable broth and scrape up the browned bits from the bottom of the pan.
5. Stir in the arrowroot powder then stir in the coconut milk and the rest of the broth.
6. Bring the mixture to a simmer then stir in the herbs, salt, and pepper.
7. Simmer the soup, covered, for 15 to 20 minutes then serve hot.

Creamy Cucumber Dill Salad

Servings: 4 to 6

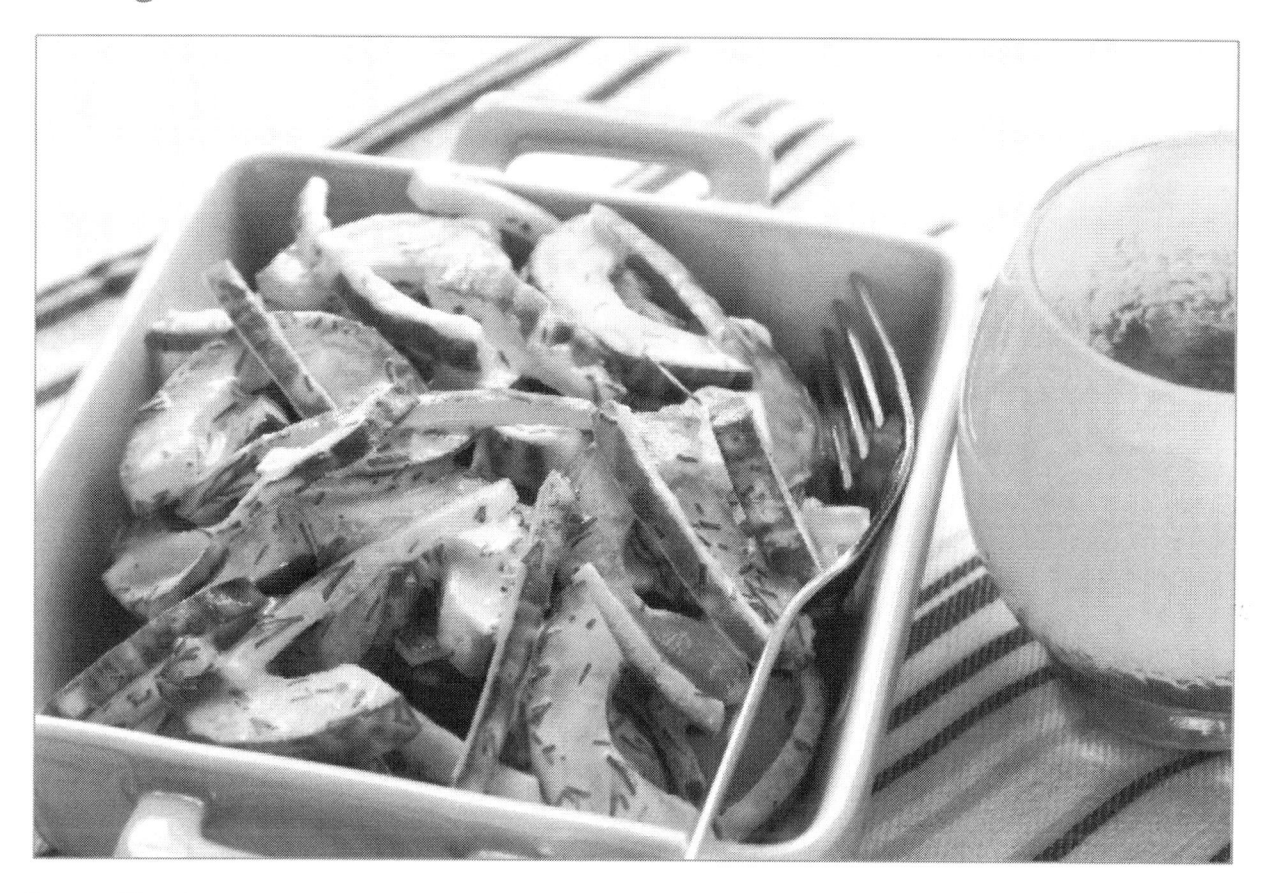

Ingredients:

- 2 large seedless cucumbers
- 1 small red onion, sliced thin
- ¼ cup canned coconut milk
- 2 tablespoons fresh chopped dill
- 1 tablespoon honey
- Salt and pepper to taste

Instructions:

1. Slice the cucumbers very thin and place them in a large bowl.
2. Add the sliced red onion and set aside.

3. Whisk together the coconut milk, dill, honey, salt, and pepper in a separate bowl.

4. Toss the dressing with the cucumber and onions to coat.

5. Chill the salad until ready to serve.

Lamb and Root Vegetable Stew

Servings: 4 to 6

Ingredients:

- 1 tablespoon coconut oil
- 2 large carrots, peeled and sliced
- 2 medium turnips, peeled and sliced
- 1 large parsnip, peeled and sliced
- 1 large sweet potato, peeled and chopped
- 1 large yellow onion, chopped
- 1 pound lamb shank, chopped
- 2 (14-ounce) cans diced tomatoes
- 4 cups beef stock (low sodium)
- 1 teaspoon fresh chopped rosemary
- ½ teaspoon fresh chopped thyme
- Salt and pepper

Instructions:

1. Heat the oil in a large saucepan over medium-high heat.
2. Add the vegetables and cook for 4 to 5 minutes until lightly browned.
3. Stir in the lamb along with the tomatoes, stock, and seasonings.
4. Bring the mixture to a boil then reduce heat and simmer, covered, for one hour – stir every 15 minutes.
5. Uncover the pot and simmer for another 45 minutes then serve hot.

Mango Walnut Salad with Pecans

Servings: 4

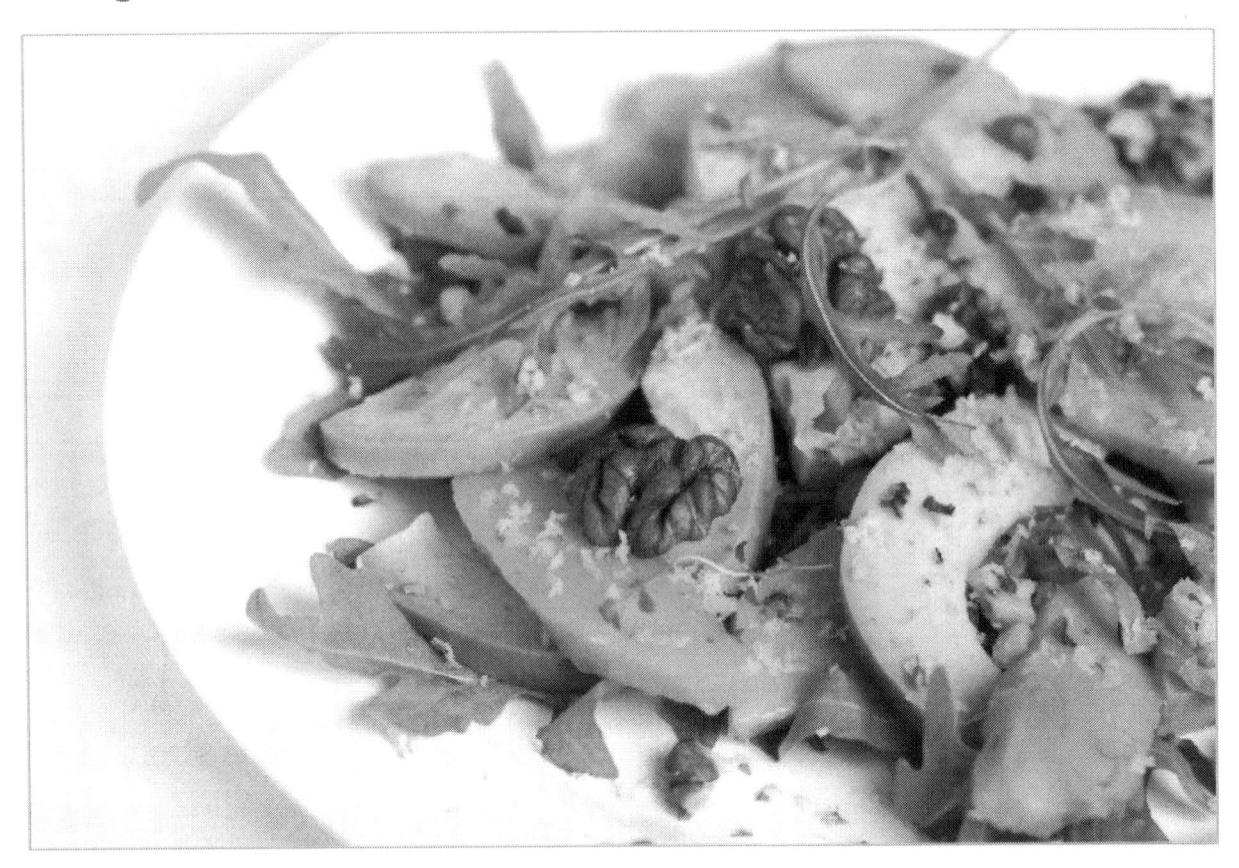

Ingredients:

- 5 cups fresh spring greens
- 2 small ripe avocadoes, pitted and sliced thin
- 1 large mango, pitted and sliced thin
- 1 cup whole toasted pecans
- ¼ cup olive oil
- 2 tablespoons fresh lemon juice
- ½ teaspoon Dijon mustard
- Salt and pepper

Instructions:

1. Place the spring greens in a large salad bowl.

2. Add the sliced avocado and mango then toss to combine.

3. Divide among four salad plates and top each salad with pecans.

4. Whisk together the remaining ingredients in a small bowl then drizzle over the salads to serve.

Easy Chicken and Vegetable Soup

Servings: 6 to 8

Ingredients:

- 1 tablespoon olive oil
- 2 cups cooked chicken breast, chopped
- 1 medium yellow onion, chopped
- 1 small leek, sliced thin (white and light green parts only)
- 8 cups low sodium chicken stock
- 2 large carrots, peeled and sliced
- 1 medium zucchini, sliced
- 1 large stalk celery, sliced
- 1 red pepper, diced
- 1 cup diced tomatoes
- ¼ cup fresh chopped parsley
- 1 teaspoon fresh chopped thyme
- ½ teaspoon fresh chopped tarragon
- Salt and pepper

Instructions:

1. Heat the oil in a large stockpot over medium heat.
2. Add the chicken, onions, and leeks and cook for 4 to 5 minutes.
3. Stir in the remaining ingredients and bring to a boil.
4. Reduce heat and simmer for 20 minutes until the vegetables are tender and the chicken heated through.

5. Season with salt and pepper to taste and serve hot.

Spiced Pumpkin Soup

Servings: 4 to 6

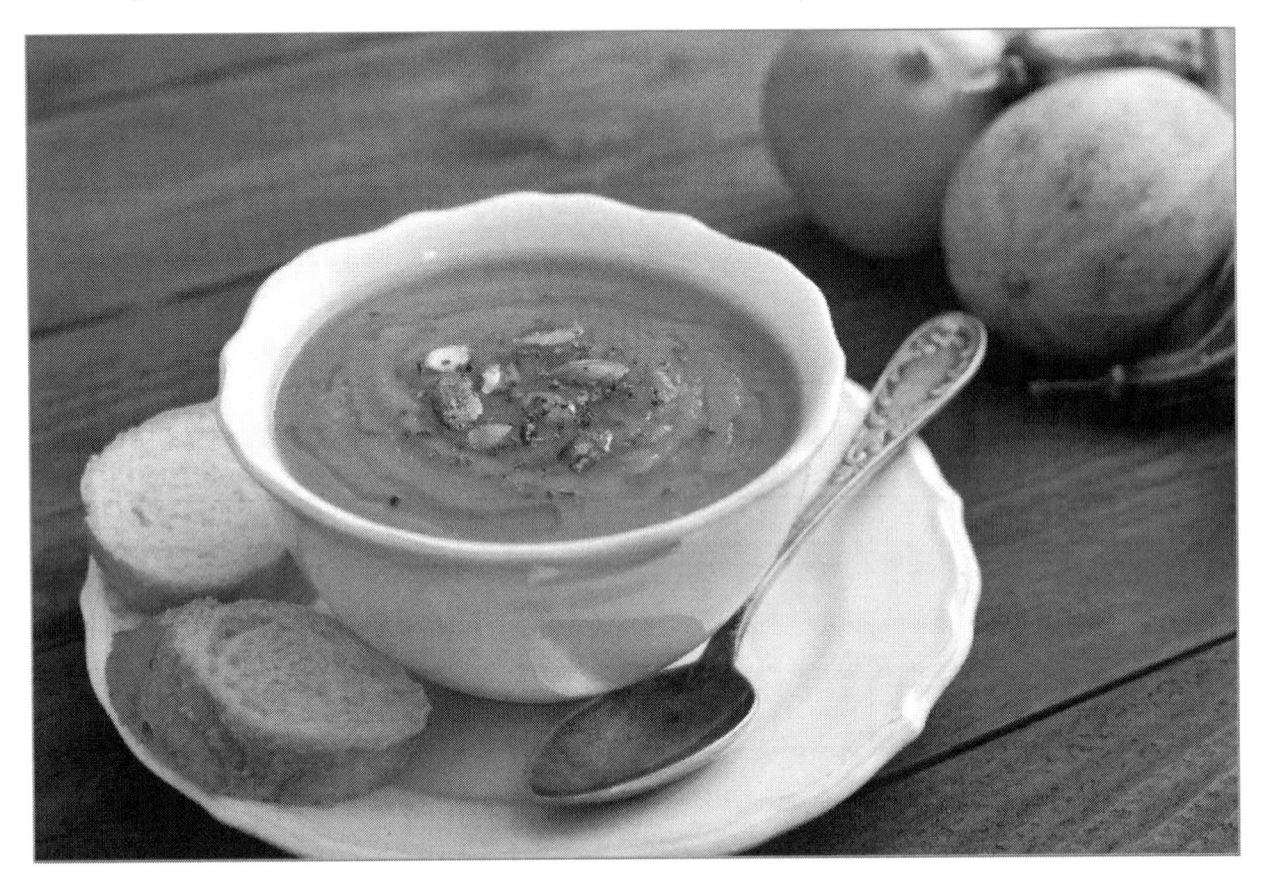

Ingredients:

- 2 tablespoons coconut oil, divided
- 6 cups chopped pumpkin
- 1 large white onion, chopped
- 1 tablespoon fresh grated ginger
- 1 teaspoon minced garlic
- 1 teaspoon ground cinnamon
- ¼ teaspoon ground nutmeg
- Salt and pepper to taste
- 4 cups vegetable stock (low sodium)

Instructions:

1. Heat 1 tablespoon oil in a large saucepan over medium heat.
2. Add the pumpkin and sauté for 6 to 8 minutes until browned.
3. Spoon the squash into a bowl and reheat the skillet with the remaining oil.
4. Add the onions, garlic, ginger, cinnamon, nutmeg, salt and pepper.
5. Cook for 4 to 6 minutes until the onions are translucent.
6. Add the pumpkin back to the pot along with the chicken stock.
7. Bring to a boil then reduce heat and simmer, covered, for 45 minutes.
8. Turn off the heat and puree the soup using an immersion blender until smooth.
9. Spoon into bowls and serve hot.

Dinner Recipes

Rosemary Roasted Chicken

Servings: 4 to 6

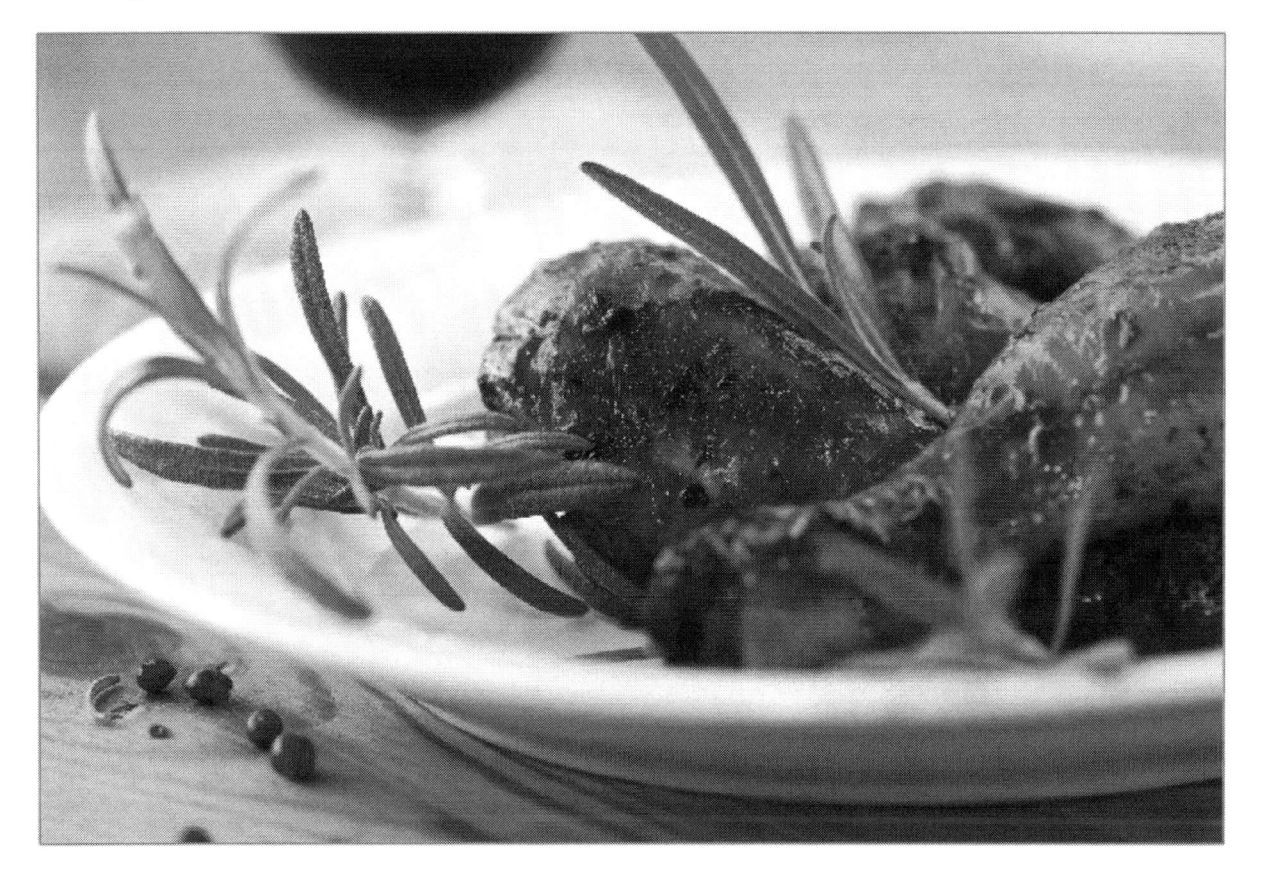

Ingredients:

- 2 to 3 pounds bone-in chicken drumsticks and thighs
- 2 tablespoons olive oil
- Salt and pepper
- 1 large yellow onion, quartered
- 1 large sweet potato, chopped coarsely
- 1 cup broccoli florets
- 1 cup cauliflower florets
- 1 cup baby carrots
- 1 red pepper, cored and chopped

- 1 green pepper, cored and chopped
- 1 tablespoon fresh chopped rosemary
- 1 teaspoon fresh chopped thyme
- ¼ cup chicken broth (low sodium)

Instructions:

1. Preheat the oven to 400°F.
2. Season the chicken with salt and pepper to taste.
3. Heat the oil in a large skillet over medium-high heat.
4. Add the chicken in batches and cook until evenly browned, turning as needed.
5. Combine the vegetables in a large bowl and toss to coat with oil, rosemary, and thyme.
6. Spread the vegetables in a large rectangular glass baking dish and arrange the chicken on top of it.
7. Drizzle with chicken broth then roast for 50 to 60 minutes until the chicken is cooked through and the vegetables tender.

Thai Coconut Vegetable Curry

Servings: 4

Ingredients:

- 1 tablespoon coconut oil
- 1 medium yellow onion, chopped
- 1 tablespoon fresh grated ginger
- 1 tablespoon fresh minced garlic
- 1 cup sliced carrots
- 2 bell peppers, cored and chopped
- 2 tablespoons Thai curry paste
- 1 (14-ounce) can coconut milk (full fat)
- ½ cup vegetable broth
- 2 cups fresh chopped kale
- Salt, to taste

Instructions:

1. Heat the oil in a large skillet over medium heat.
2. Add the onion and cook until translucent – about 4 to 5 minutes.
3. Stir in the ginger and garlic and cook for another 30 seconds.
4. Add the carrots and bell peppers – cook for 4 to 5 minutes until tender, stirring occasionally.
5. Stir in the curry paste and cook for 2 minutes.
6. Add the coconut milk, vegetable broth, and kale then stir well.

7. Bring to a boil then reduce heat and simmer for 5 to 10 minutes until the vegetables are tender – stir as needed.

8. Season the curry with salt to taste and serve hot.

Herb-Roasted Pork Tenderloin

Servings: 6 to 8

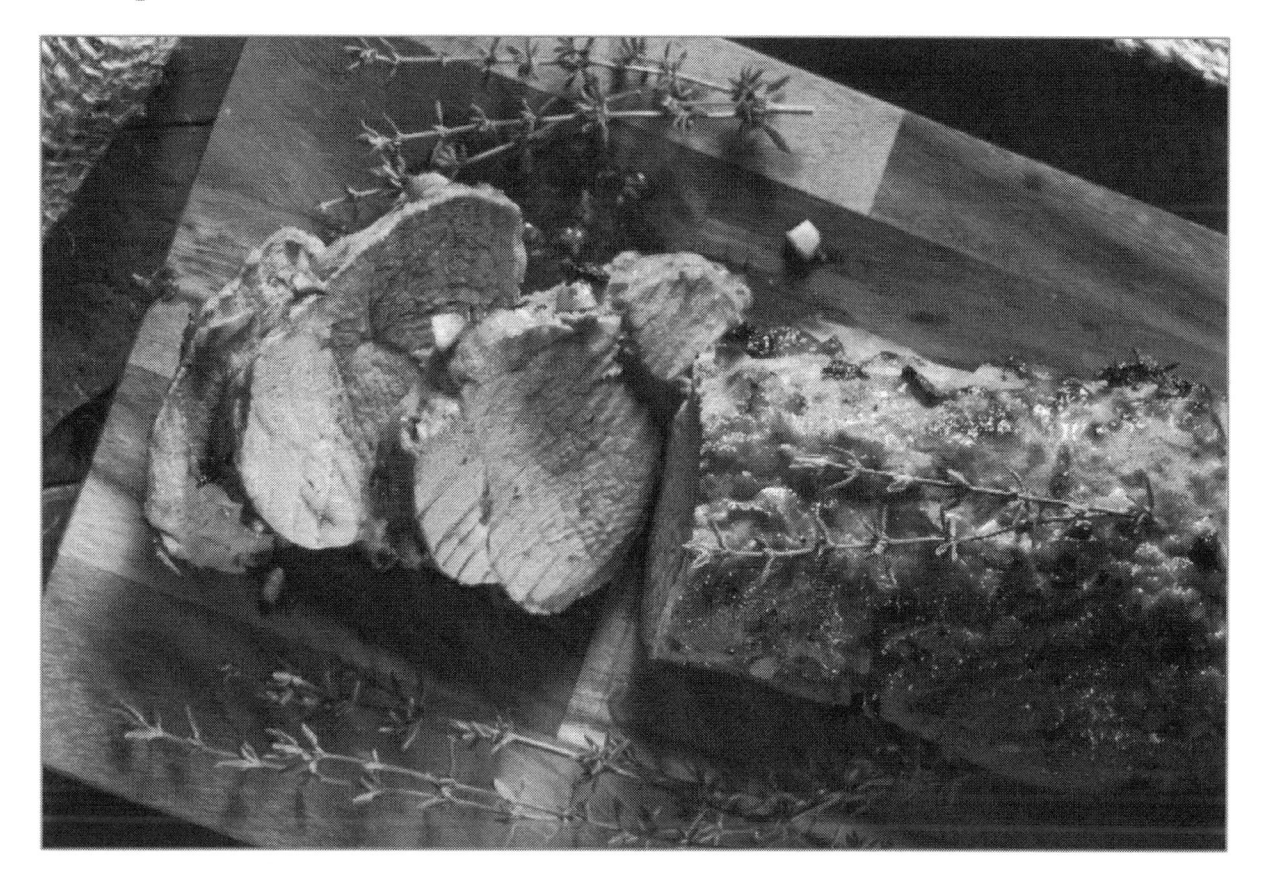

Ingredients:

- 1 (4-pound) boneless pork tenderloin
- Salt and pepper
- 2 tablespoons olive oil
- 4 shallots, sliced very thin
- 3 tablespoons Dijon mustard
- 2 tablespoons minced garlic
- 1 tablespoon fresh chopped rosemary
- 1 tablespoon fresh chopped thyme
- 1 tablespoon fresh chopped sage

Instructions:

1. Preheat the oven to 350°F.
2. Use a paper towel to pat the pork tenderloin dry then season generously with salt and pepper.
3. Heat the oil in a large skillet over medium-high heat then add the pork and brown on all sides.
4. Combine the sliced shallots, mustard, garlic, and herbs in a bowl.
5. Place the pork on a rack in a roasting pan and spread the herb mixture over it.
6. Roast the pork for 1 hour then keep cooking, checking every 5 minutes, until the internal temperature reads 140°F to 145°F.
7. Transfer the pork to a cutting board and let rest for 15 minutes before slicing.

Balsamic Grilled Salmon

Servings: 4

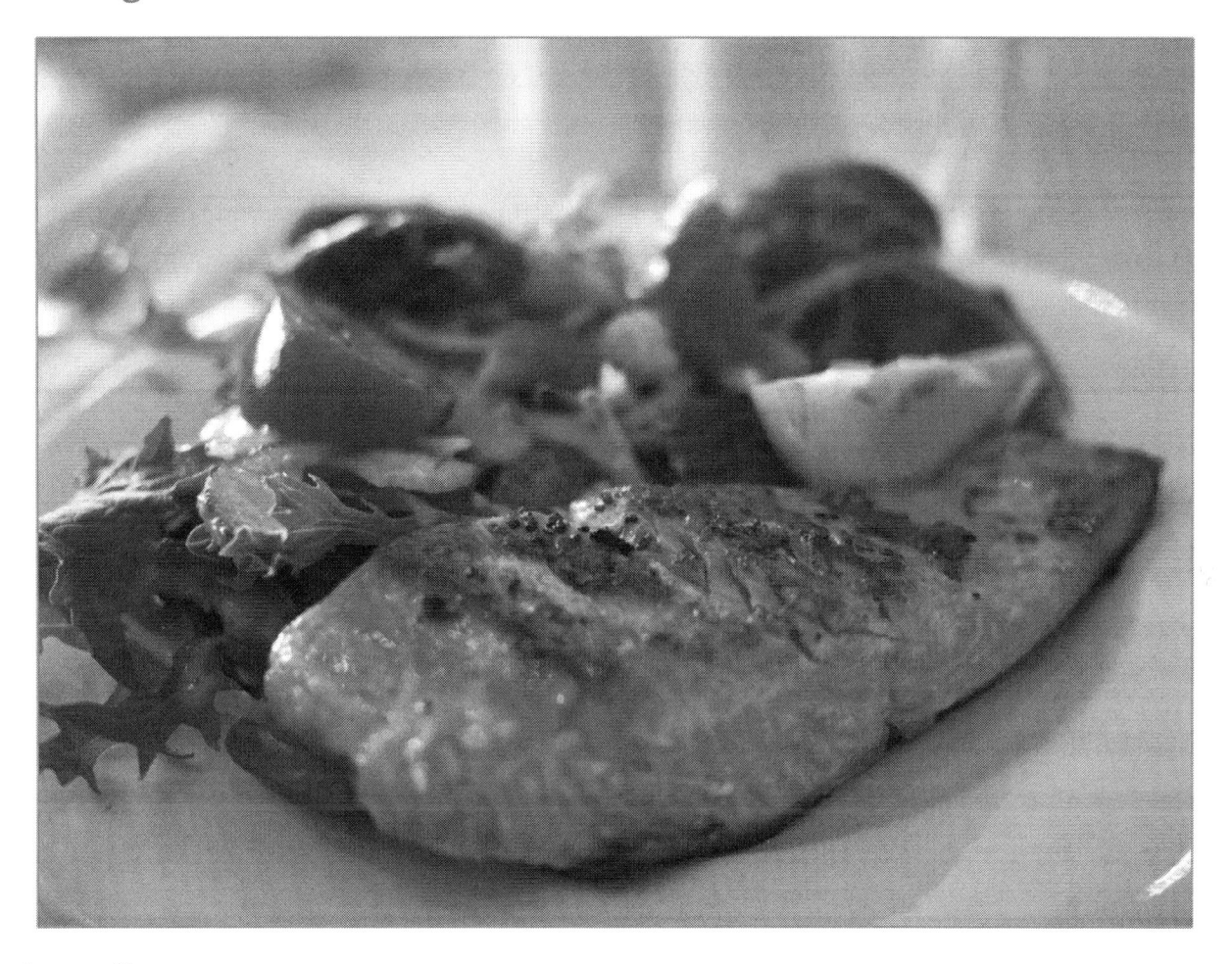

Ingredients:

- Olive oil, as needed
- 3 tablespoons honey
- 2 tablespoons Dijon mustard
- 2 tablespoons balsamic vinegar
- ½ teaspoon salt
- ¼ teaspoon black pepper
- 4 (6-ounce) boneless salmon fillets
- Lemon wedges

Instructions:

1. Preheat a grill to medium-high heat and brush the grates with olive oil.

2. Whisk together the honey, Dijon mustard, balsamic vinegar, salt and pepper in a small bowl.

3. Brush the mixture over the salmon fillets and place them on the grill.

4. Cover the grill and cook for 2 to 3 minutes on each side until the flesh flakes easily with a fork.

5. Drizzle with extra glaze, if desired, and serve with lemon wedges.

Slow Cooker Pulled Pork

Servings: 8 to 10

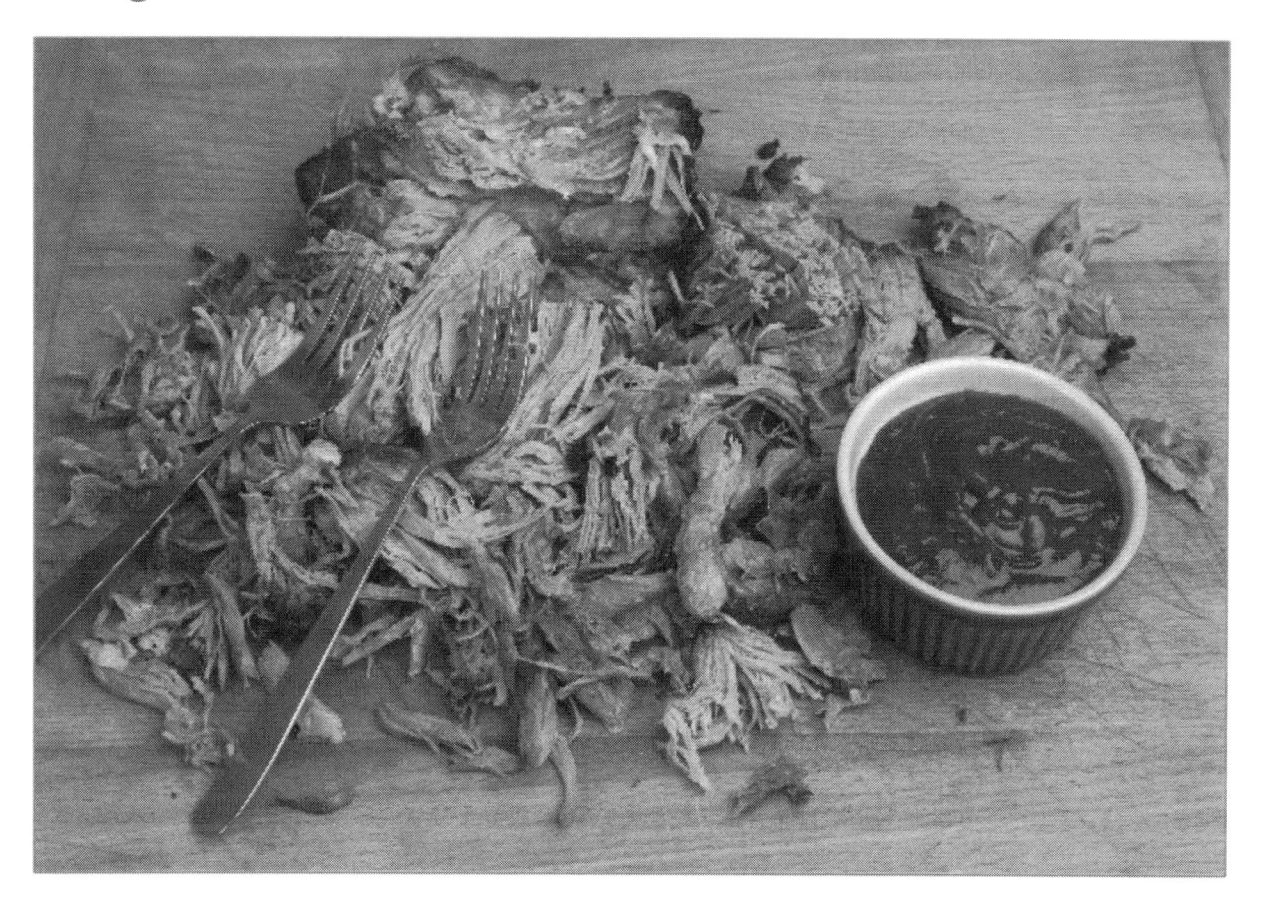

Ingredients:

- 4 pounds boneless pork shoulder
- ¼ cup smoked paprika
- 2 tablespoons chili powder
- 2 tablespoons ground cumin
- 1 tablespoon salt
- 1 tablespoon white pepper
- 1 to 2 cups barbecue sauce

Instructions:

1. Combine the paprika, chili powder, cumin, salt and pepper in a small bowl.
2. Rub the spice mixture into the pork shoulder on all sides.
3. Wrap the pork in two layers of plastic and chill for at least 4 hours.
4. Place the unwrapped pork shoulder in a slow cooker then pour in the water.
5. Cover and cook on low heat for 8 to 10 hours until the pork is very tender.
6. Transfer the pork to a cutting board and shred it with two forks.
7. Return the pork to the slow cooker with the juices and toss with your favorite paleo barbecue sauce.

Veggie-Stuffed Zucchini Boats

Servings: 4

Ingredients:

- 4 medium zucchini
- 1 small red pepper, cored and diced
- ½ small yellow onion, diced
- 3 cloves minced garlic
- 1 cup diced tomatoes
- Salt and pepper
- 2 large eggs, whisked well
- ¼ cup almond flour

Instructions:

1. Preheat the oven to 400°F and line a baking sheet with foil.
2. Slice the zucchini in half lengthwise then use a spoon to scoop out the flesh.
3. Chop the zucchini flesh into a bowl and stir in the chopped peppers, onions, and garlic.
4. Heat the oil in a large skillet over medium heat and add the chopped vegetables.
5. Cook for 8 to 10 minutes, stirring often, then add the tomatoes and cook for 2 minutes more.
6. Turn off the heat and season the mixture with salt and pepper then spoon into a bowl.

7. Stir in the eggs and almond flour then spoon the mixture into the zucchini shells and place them on the baking sheet.

8. Bake for 25 minutes then remove from oven and cool 10 minutes before serving.

Baked Haddock with Mango Salsa

Servings: 4

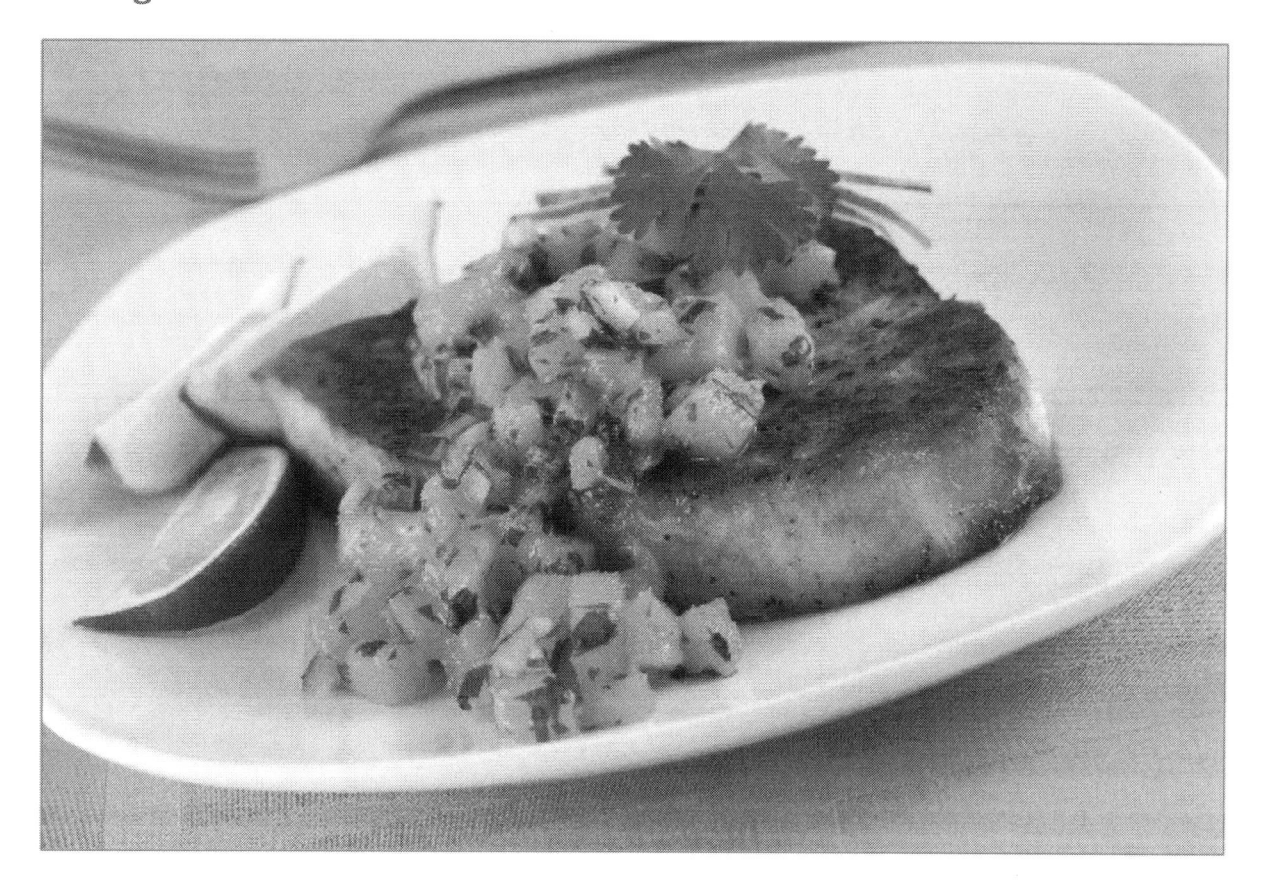

Ingredients:

- 4 (6-ounce) boneless haddock fillets
- Salt and pepper
- 1 medium ripe mango, pitted and chopped
- ¼ cup diced red onion
- ¼ cup fresh chopped cilantro
- 1 tablespoon fresh lime juice

Instructions:

1. Preheat the oven to 375°F.

2. Brush the haddock fillets with olive oil and season lightly with salt and pepper.

3. Place the fillets on a baking sheet and bake for 10 to 15 minutes until the flesh flakes easily with a fork.

4. Meanwhile, combine the remaining ingredients in a food processor.

5. Pulse until finely chopped then spoon the salsa over the fish to serve.

Seared Scallops with Herb Butter

Servings: 4

Ingredients:

- 1 tablespoon coconut oil
- 1 ¼ pounds large sea scallops, rinsed and patted dry
- Salt and pepper
- 3 tablespoons grass-fed butter, chopped
- 2 tablespoons fresh chopped herbs (your choice)
- 1 tablespoon fresh lemon juice

Instructions:

1. Heat the oil in a large skillet over medium-high heat.
2. Lightly season the scallops with salt and pepper then place them in the hot oil.
3. Sear for 2 to 3 minutes on one side until golden brown.
4. Carefully turn the scallops then add the butter and herbs to the skillet.
5. Cook for 2 to 3 minutes until the scallops are just cooked through.
6. Drizzle with lemon juice and serve hot.

Meatloaf with BBQ Sauce

Servings: 6 to 8

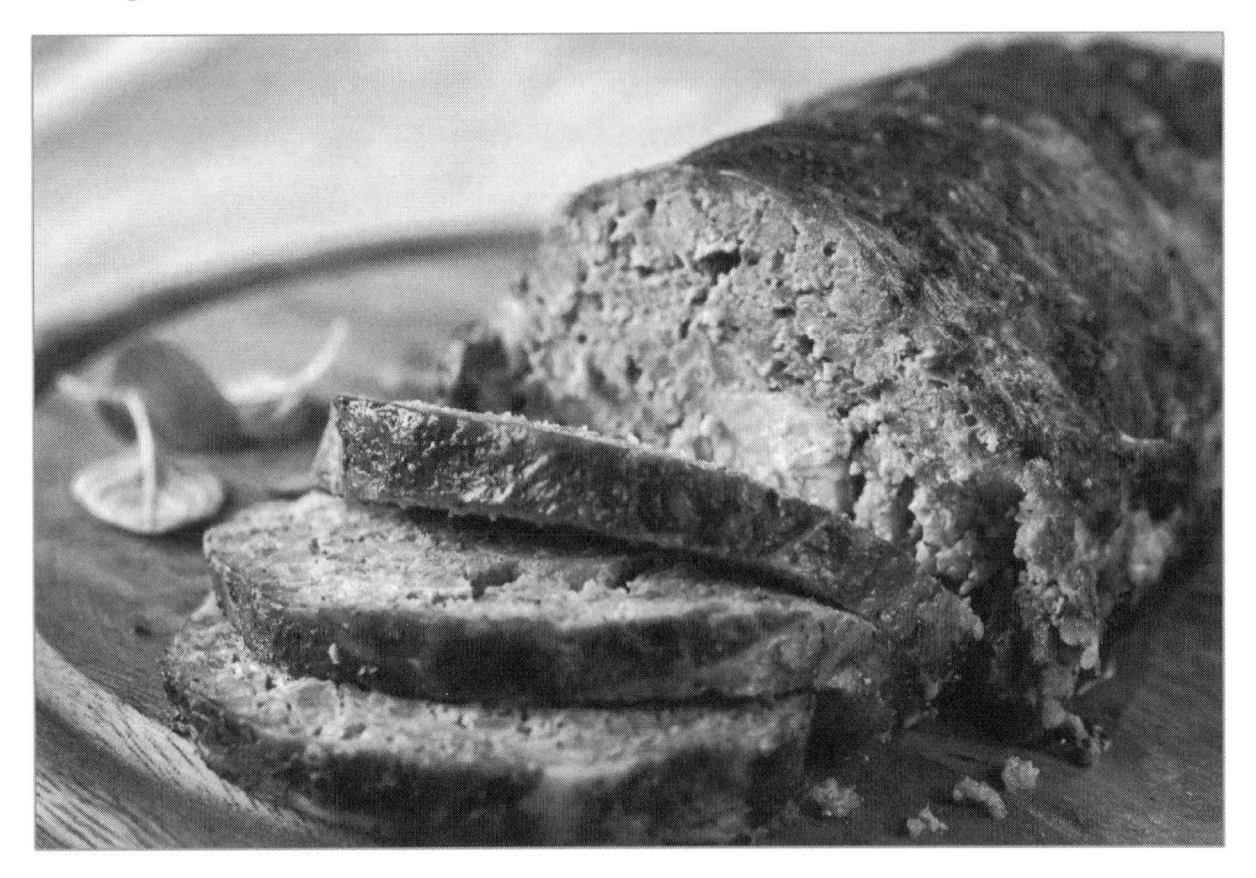

Ingredients:

- 1 tablespoon olive oil
- 1 small yellow onion, chopped
- 3 cloves minced garlic
- 1 teaspoon fresh chopped oregano
- 1 teaspoon fresh chopped thyme
- Salt and pepper
- 1 pound lean ground beef
- 1 pound lean ground turkey breast
- 3 large eggs, whisked

- ½ cup almond flour
- ½ cup paleo barbecue sauce

Instructions:

1. Preheat the oven to 350°F.
2. Heat the oil in a small saucepan over medium heat until tender.
3. Stir in the onions, garlic, oregano, thyme, salt and pepper then remove from heat.
4. Place the ground beef and turkey in a large mixing bowl.
5. Add the eggs and almond flour, mixing it together by hand.
6. Work the vegetable mixture into the meat then shape it into a loaf and place it on a roasting pan.
7. Pour the barbecue sauce over the meatloaf.
8. Bake for 1 hour and 5 to 15 minutes until the internal temperature reaches 155°F.
9. Remove the meatloaf from the oven and let rest 10 minutes before serving.

Herb-Crusted Lamb Chops

Servings: 4 to 6

Ingredients:

- 2 pounds bone-in lamb chops
- Salt and pepper
- 3 tablespoons olive oil
- 2 tablespoons minced garlic
- ¼ cup fresh chopped parsley
- ½ teaspoon fresh chopped rosemary
- ½ teaspoon fresh chopped thyme
- Coconut oil, as needed

Instructions:

1. Pat the lamb chops dry with paper towel and season with salt and pepper.
2. Whisk together the olive oil, garlic, parsley, rosemary, and thyme in a small bowl.
3. Arrange the lamb chops in a shallow dish and pour the marinade over them, turning to coat.
4. Cover and chill for 6 to 12 hours.
5. Take the lamb chops out of the refrigerator 30 minutes prior to cooking.
6. Heat some coconut oil in a large skillet over high heat.
7. Add the lamb chops and cook for 3 to 4 minutes on each side until seared.

Slow Cooker Chicken Cacciatore

Servings: 5 to 6

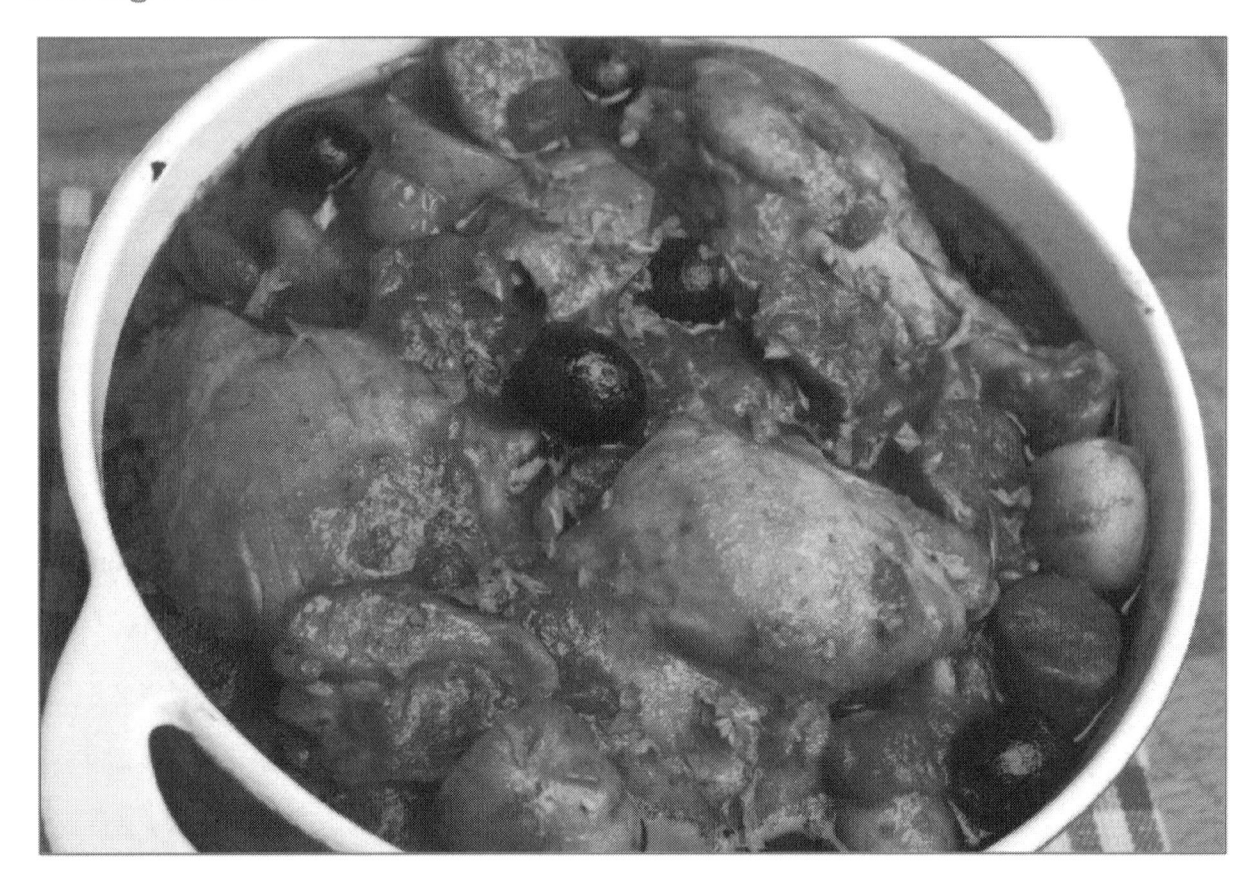

Ingredients:

- ➢ 1 tablespoon olive oil
- ➢ 1 large yellow onion, chopped
- ➢ ¼ cup tomato paste
- ➢ 1 tablespoon minced garlic
- ➢ 1 ½ teaspoons dried oregano
- ➢ ½ teaspoon dried thyme
- ➢ ¼ teaspoon red pepper flakes
- ➢ 1 (14.5-ounce) can diced tomatoes
- ➢ 2 pounds sliced mushrooms

- ➤ 1 cup pitted black olives
- ➤ ½ cup low-sodium chicken stock
- ➤ 2 pounds chicken thighs and drumsticks

Instructions:

1. Heat the oil in a large skillet over medium heat.
2. Add the onions and cook for 5 to 6 minutes until translucent.
3. Stir in the tomato paste, garlic, and spices and cook for 2 minutes.
4. Spread the mixture in the bottom of the slow cooker.
5. Add the tomatoes, mushrooms, olives, and chicken stock.
6. Season the chicken with salt and pepper and place it in the slow cooker.
7. Cover and cook on low heat for 4 to 6 hours until the chicken is cooked through.

Zucchini Pasta and Meatballs

Servings: 4

Ingredients:

- 2 cups pasta sauce
- 3 large zucchini
- 1 pound lean ground beef
- 1 pound lean ground turkey
- 1 large egg, whisked
- ½ cup almond flour
- 2 ½ tablespoons coconut aminos
- 1 tablespoon Italian seasoning
- Salt to taste

Instructions:

1. Preheat the oven to 400°F and line a baking sheet with foil.
2. Place the pasta sauce in a saucepan and warm over medium heat.
3. Use a vegetable peeler or mandolin to slice the zucchini into noodle-like strips or threads.
4. Set the zucchini noodles aside while you prepare the meatballs.
5. Combine the beef, turkey, egg, almond flour, coconut aminos, Italian seasoning and salt in a bowl, mixing by hand.
6. Shape the mixture into 1-inch balls and arrange them on the baking sheet.
7. Bake for 18 to 22 minutes until the meatballs are cooked through.

8. Heat some oil in a large skillet over medium heat.

9. Add the zucchini and cook until just heated through then serve with the meatballs and pasta sauce.

Chicken Tikka Masala

Servings: 4 to 6

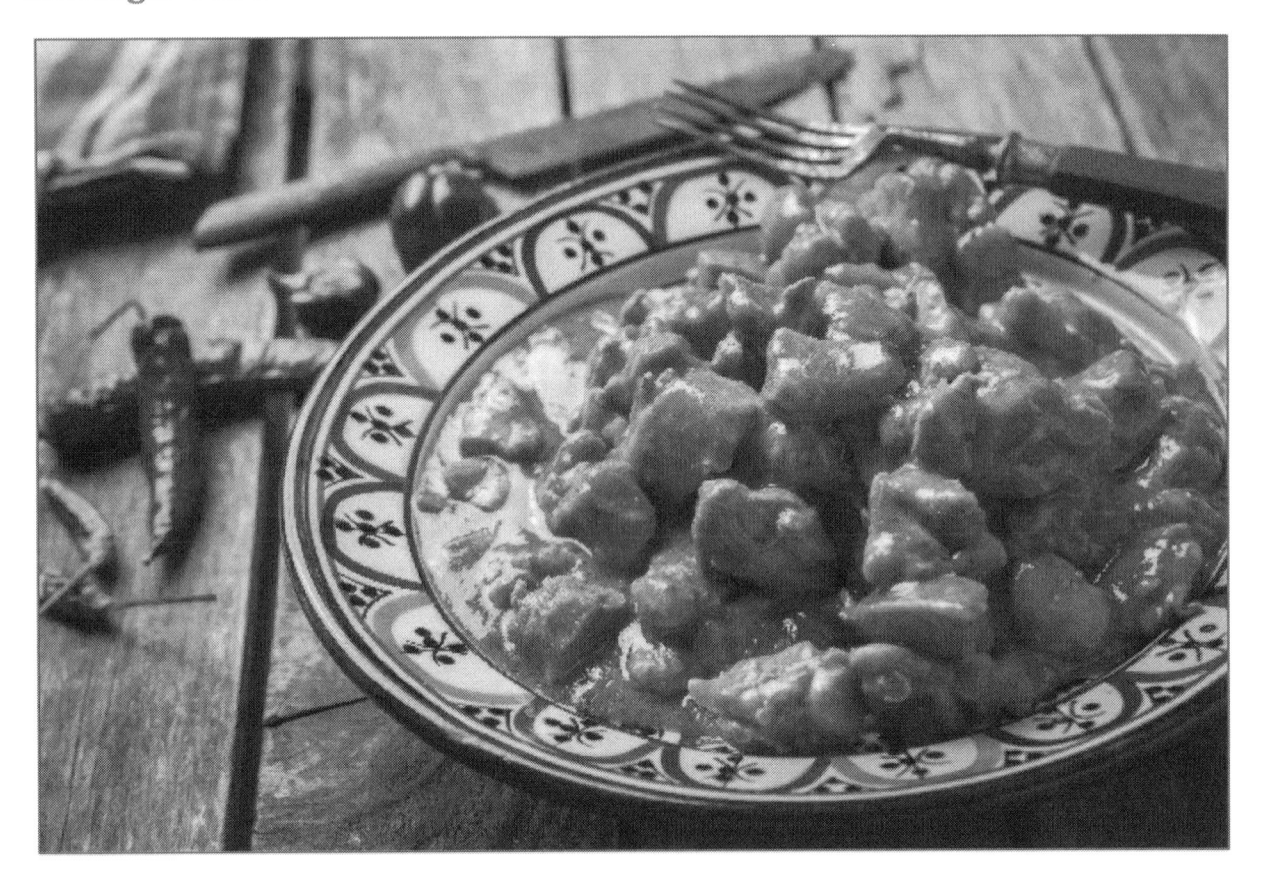

Ingredients:

- ½ cup raw cashews
- 3 pounds boneless chicken thighs, chopped
- 1 tablespoon minced garlic
- 3 tablespoons garam masala
- 2 ½ teaspoons salt
- 1 ½ teaspoons ground ginger
- ½ teaspoon paprika
- ½ teaspoon cayenne
- 2 cups tomato puree

- 1 medium yellow onion, chopped

Instructions:

1. Place the cashews in a bowl and add enough water to cover them.
2. Cover the bowl with plastic and set aside.
3. Spread the chicken in a slow cooker and sprinkle with the garlic and spices.
4. Add the tomato puree and onions then cover and cook on low heat for 6 hours.
5. During the last 15 minutes of cooking, drain the cashews and put them in a blender with ¼ cup water.
6. Blend the cashews until smooth then stir it into the slow cooker.
7. Allow the chicken tikka masala to cook for another 5 minutes until heated through then serve hot.

Sausage Sweet Potato Chili

Servings: 4 to 6

Ingredients:

- 6 slices uncooked bacon
- 2 tablespoons olive oil
- 2 large sweet potatoes, peeled and chopped
- 1 small yellow onion, chopped
- 2 cloves minced garlic
- 1 pound ground chorizo sausage
- 1 (14.5-ounce) can roasted tomatoes
- 1 cup tomato sauce
- 1 tablespoon chili powder
- 1 teaspoon ground cumin
- ½ teaspoon smoked paprika
- Pinch cayenne

Instructions:

1. Cook the bacon in a skillet over medium-high heat until crisp.
2. Drain the bacon on paper towels then chop coarsely.
3. In a separate skillet, heat the oil over medium heat.
4. Add the sweet potatoes then cook, covered, for 2 minutes.
5. Remove the lid and cook for 4 to 5 minutes, stirring occasionally, until they are just tender.
6. Add the onions and garlic and cook for 2 minutes.

7. Stir in the chorizo, breaking it up into chunks as it cooks, until evenly browned.

8. Add the tomatoes, tomato sauce, and spices then stir well.

9. Simmer over medium heat until it starts to boil then reduce heat to low and cook for 5 minutes then serve the chili hot with chopped bacon.

Slow Cooker Balsamic Roast Beef

Servings: 4 to 6

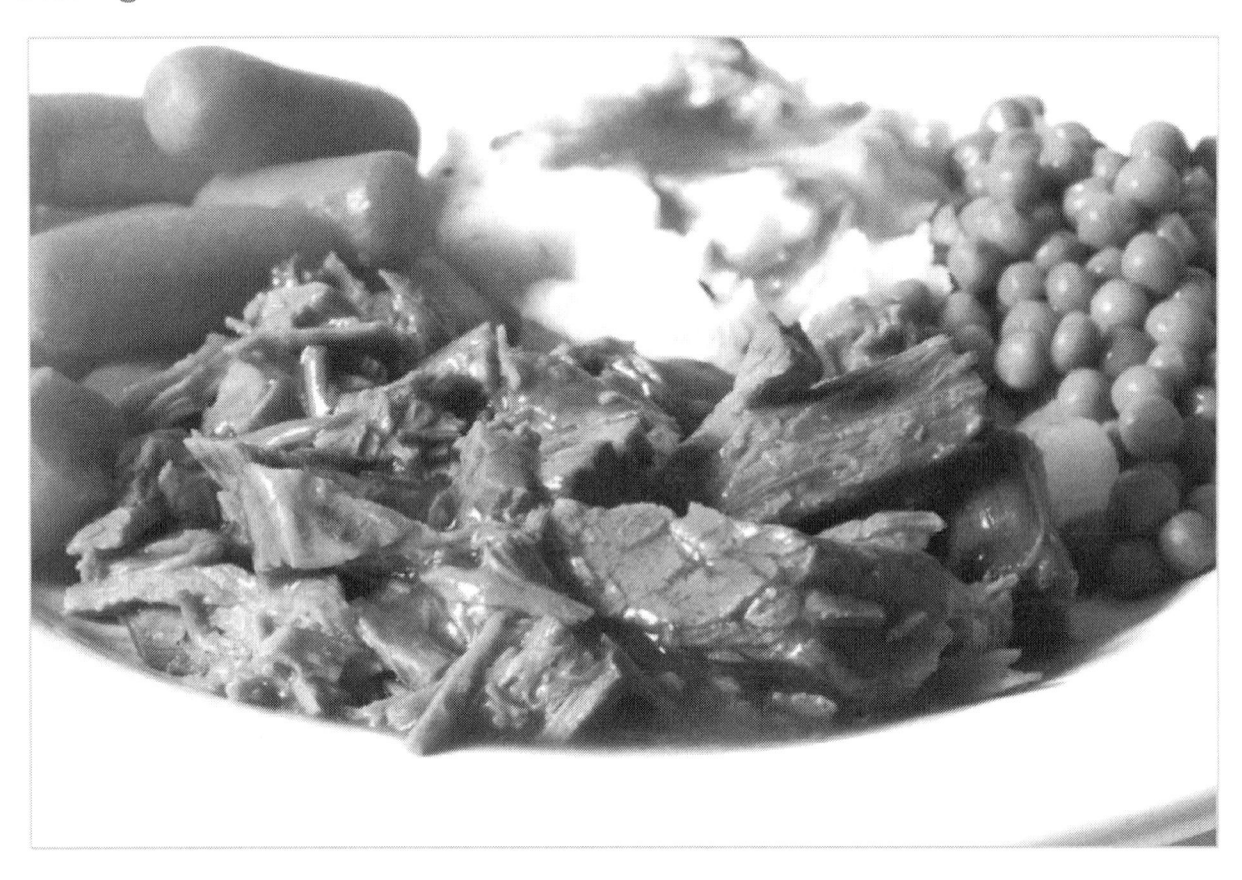

Ingredients:

- 3 pounds boneless beef chuck roast
- Salt and pepper
- 2 tablespoons coconut oil
- 1 large yellow onion, sliced
- 1 tablespoon minced garlic
- 2 cups beef stock
- ½ cup balsamic vinegar
- 2 tablespoons fresh chopped rosemary
- 3 large sweet potatoes, chopped

- ➢ 4 medium carrots, peeled and sliced

Instructions:

1. Season the chuck roast with salt and pepper.
2. Heat the oil in a large skillet over medium-high heat.
3. Add the roast and cook until it is browned on all sides, about 2 to 3 minutes per side.
4. Place the roast in a slow cooker and add the onion and garlic.
5. Drizzle in the beef stock and balsamic vinegar then sprinkle with rosemary.
6. Cover and cook on low heat for 6 hours.
7. Add the sweet potatoes and carrots then cook, covered, on high for 3 hours until the meat is very tender.
8. Remove the roast to a cutting board and cover loosely with foil.
9. Use a slotted spoon to remove the vegetables to a bowl then pour the cooking liquid into a saucepan.
10. Bring the liquid to a slow boil and simmer until it thickens.
11. Slice the roast and serve with the vegetables, drizzled in sauce.

Cajun Chicken and Veggies

Servings: 4

Ingredients:

- Olive oil, as needed
- 3 pounds bone-in chicken thighs
- 1 tablespoon paprika
- 2 teaspoons garlic powder
- 2 teaspoons salt
- 1 ½ teaspoons dried oregano
- 1 ½ teaspoons dried thyme
- 1 teaspoon onion powder
- 1 teaspoon black pepper
- ½ teaspoon cayenne
- 2 pounds sweet potatoes, chopped
- 1 red pepper, cored and chopped
- 1 small red onion, chopped

Instructions:

1. Rub the olive oil into the chicken and place it on a rimmed baking sheet.
2. Combine the spices in a small bowl then rub the mixture into both sides of the chicken.
3. Place the sweet potatoes in a large bowl and drizzle with oil then toss with some of the spice mixture.

4. Spread the sweet potatoes on the baking sheet around the chicken and roast for 30 minutes.

5. Sprinkle on the red pepper and onions and roast for another 10 to 15 minutes until the chicken is cooked through.

6. Serve the chicken hot with the roasted vegetables.

Easy Garlic Shrimp

Servings: 4

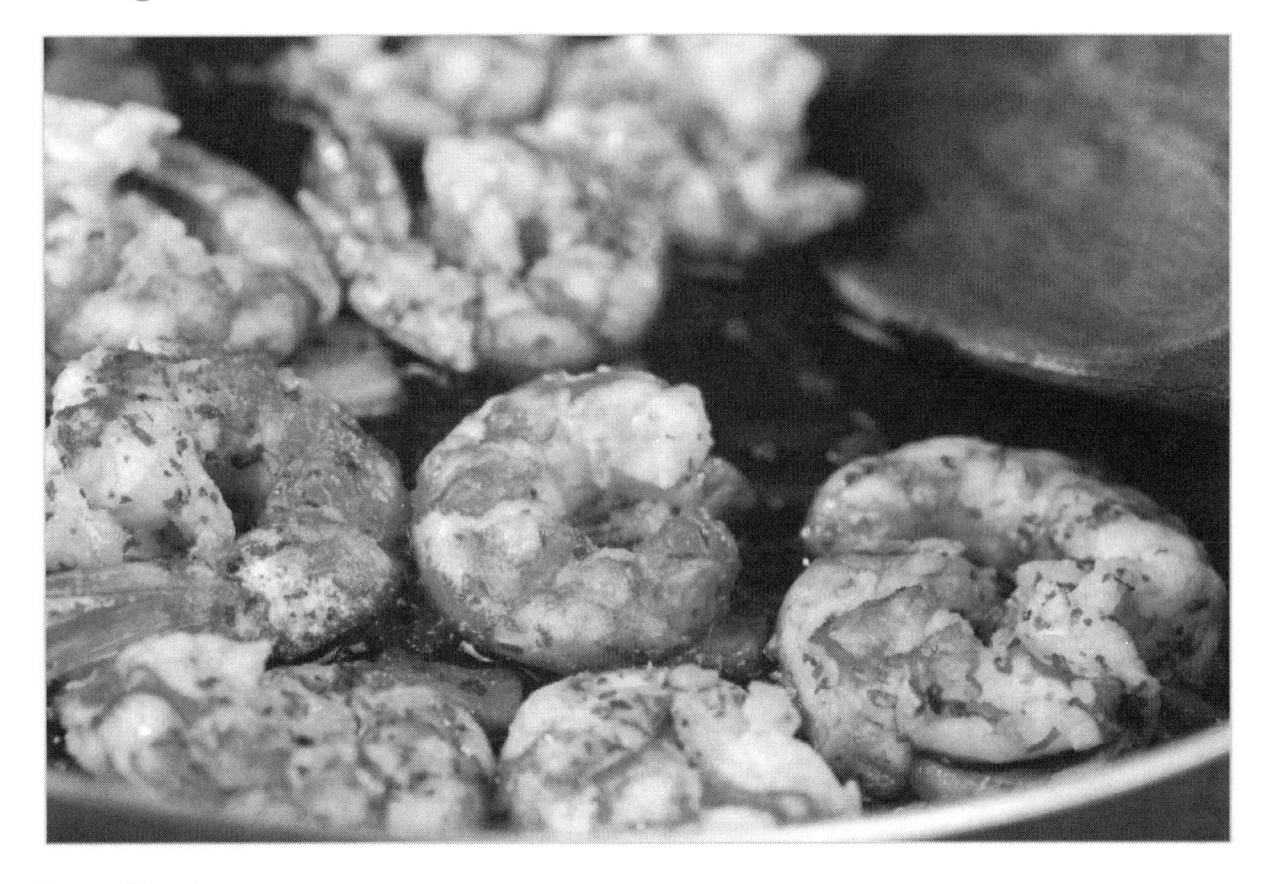

Ingredients:

- 3 tablespoons olive oil
- 2 tablespoons minced garlic
- 1 ¼ pound large uncooked shrimp, peeled and deveined
- 1 teaspoon salt
- ¼ teaspoon pepper
- Paprika, as needed

Instructions:

1. Heat the oil in a large skillet over medium-low heat.
2. Add the garlic and cook for 2 to 3 minutes until softened and fragrant.

3. Place the shrimp in the skillet in a single layer then increase the heat to medium-high.

4. Season the shrimp with salt and pepper as well as a pinch of paprika.

5. Cook the shrimp for 2 to 3 minutes until the bottom half turns pink.

6. Flip the shrimp and cook for another minute or two until just opaque.

Bacon-Wrapped Turkey Breast

Servings: 6 to 8

Ingredients:

- 4 pounds boneless skinless turkey breast
- 10 to 12 slices uncooked bacon
- Salt and pepper
- 2 tablespoons olive oil

Instructions:

1. Preheat the oven to 400°F.
2. Cut the turkey breast into chunks then season with salt and pepper.
3. Wrap each piece of turkey in a slice of bacon.
4. Heat the oil in a large cast-iron skillet over medium-high heat.
5. Add the turkey to the skillet and cook for 2 minutes until the underside is browned.
6. Flip the turkey and transfer the skillet to the oven.
7. Cook for 10 to 15 minutes until the turkey is cooked through and the bacon is crispy. Serve hot.

Grilled Salmon with Mango Sauce

Servings: 4

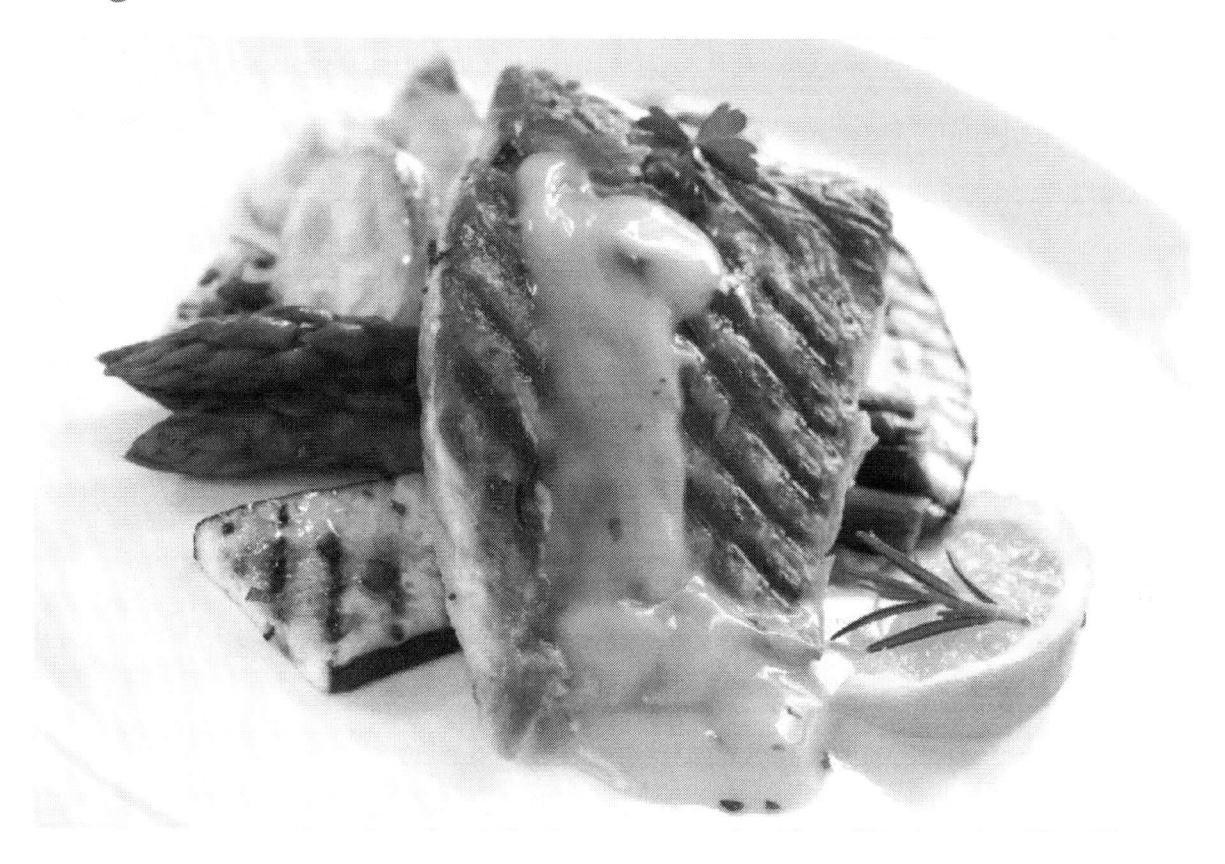

Ingredients:

- 4 (6-ounce) boneless salmon fillets
- Olive oil
- Salt and pepper
- 1 ripe mango, pitted and chopped
- ¼ cup canned coconut milk
- 2 tablespoons fresh chopped cilantro
- 1 teaspoon fresh lime juice

Instructions:

1. Preheat a grill to medium-high heat and brush the grates with olive oil.

2. Season the salmon fillets with salt and pepper then place them on the grill.

3. Cover the grill and cook for 2 to 3 minutes on each side until the flesh flakes easily with a fork.

4. While the salmon cooks, combine the remaining ingredients in a food processor or blender.

5. Blend until smooth then serve drizzled over the grilled salmon.

Lemon Chicken with Broccoli

Servings: 4 to 6

Ingredients:

- 2 tablespoons olive oil
- 4 large boneless skinless chicken breasts
- Salt and pepper
- Italian seasoning, to taste
- 1 cup low-sodium chicken broth
- ¼ cup fresh lemon juice
- 1 tablespoon minced garlic
- 1 (10-ounce) bag frozen broccoli florets
- 1 large lemon, sliced

Instructions:

1. Heat the oil in a large skillet over medium heat.
2. Season the chicken with salt, pepper, and Italian seasoning then add it to the skillet.
3. Cook for 3 to 4 minutes until the underside is browned then turn the chicken and brown on the other side.
4. Remove the chicken to a plate and reheat the skillet.
5. Add the chicken broth, lemon juice, and garlic, stirring to scrape up any browned bits from the bottom of the pan.
6. Add the chicken to the skillet along with the lemon.
7. Simmer for 5 minutes, turning the chicken halfway through.

8. Add the broccoli and cook for 5 minutes or until it is bright green and tender-crisp.

9. Adjust seasoning to taste and serve hot.

Maple BBQ Ribs

Servings: 4

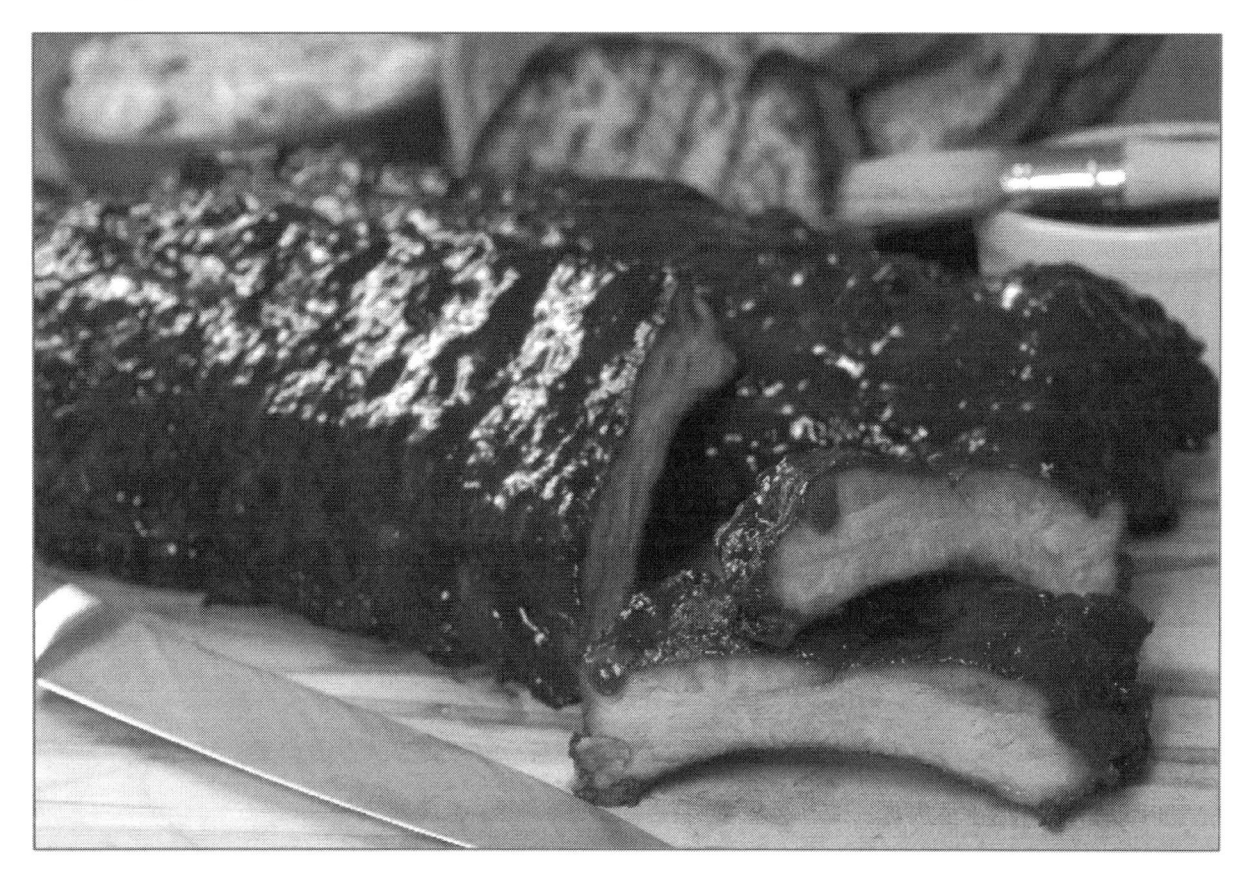

Ingredients:

- 1 tablespoon smoked paprika
- 1 tablespoon onion powder
- ½ tablespoon ground cumin
- Salt and pepper
- 4 pounds pork ribs (with bone)
- 1 tablespoon olive oil
- 1 medium white onion, minced
- 3 cloves garlic, minced
- 1 cup paleo ketchup

- ➢ 1 cup apple juice (unsweetened)
- ➢ ¼ cup maple syrup
- ➢ ¼ cup apple cider vinegar

Instructions:

1. Combine the spices in a small bowl.
2. Season the ribs with salt and pepper then spread the spice mixture over them.
3. Place the ribs in a dish and cover with plastic then chill for 2 to 12 hours.
4. Preheat the oven to 300°F. x
5. Wrap the ribs in foil and place them on a baking sheet.
6. Bake for 2 hours until the meat is very tender and falling off the bone.
7. To make the sauce, heat the oil in a saucepan over medium heat.
8. Add the onions and garlic then cook for 4 minutes.
9. Stir in the remaining ingredients and simmer for 15 to 20 minutes, stirring often.
10. When the ribs are done, brush with the sauce.
11. Increase the oven temperature to 400°F and cook the ribs for another 15 to 20 minutes, brushing with sauce every 5 minutes.
12. Just before serving, brown the ribs under the broiler.

Cilantro Lime Chicken

Servings: 4

Ingredients:

- ¼ cup olive oil
- ¼ cup fresh chopped cilantro
- 2 tablespoons lime juice
- 1 tablespoon minced garlic
- 1 teaspoon ground cumin
- ½ teaspoon red pepper flakes
- 2 pounds boneless chicken thighs
- Salt and pepper
- 2 tablespoons cooking oil

Instructions:

1. Whisk together the olive oil, cilantro, lime juice, garlic, cumin, and red pepper flakes in a bowl.
2. Place the chicken in a shallow dish and season with salt and pepper.
3. Pour the marinade over it, turning to coat, then cover and chill for up to 2 hours.
4. Preheat the oven to 375°F.
5. Melt the coconut oil in a large ovenproof skillet over medium-high heat.
6. Add the chicken and cook until browned on both sides, about 2 to 3 minutes.

7. Transfer the chicken to the oven and bake for 15 to 20 minutes until cooked through.

8. Sprinkle with cilantro and drizzle with lime juice to serve.

Curry Grilled Pork Chops

Servings: 4

Ingredients:

- 4 bone-in pork chops, 1-inch thick
- Salt and pepper
- 1 tablespoon olive oil
- 1 ½ teaspoons curry powder

Instructions:

1. Preheat the grill to high heat and brush the grates with oil.
2. Season the pork chops with salt and pepper to taste then place them in a shallow dish.
3. Whisk together the olive oil and curry powder then pour over the pork chops, turning to coat.
4. Place the pork chops on the grill and cook for 3 to 4 minutes on each side until just cooked through.
5. Remove the pork chops to a cutting board and let rest 5 minutes before serving.

Snacks & Dessert

Baked Cinnamon Apple Chips

Servings: 4

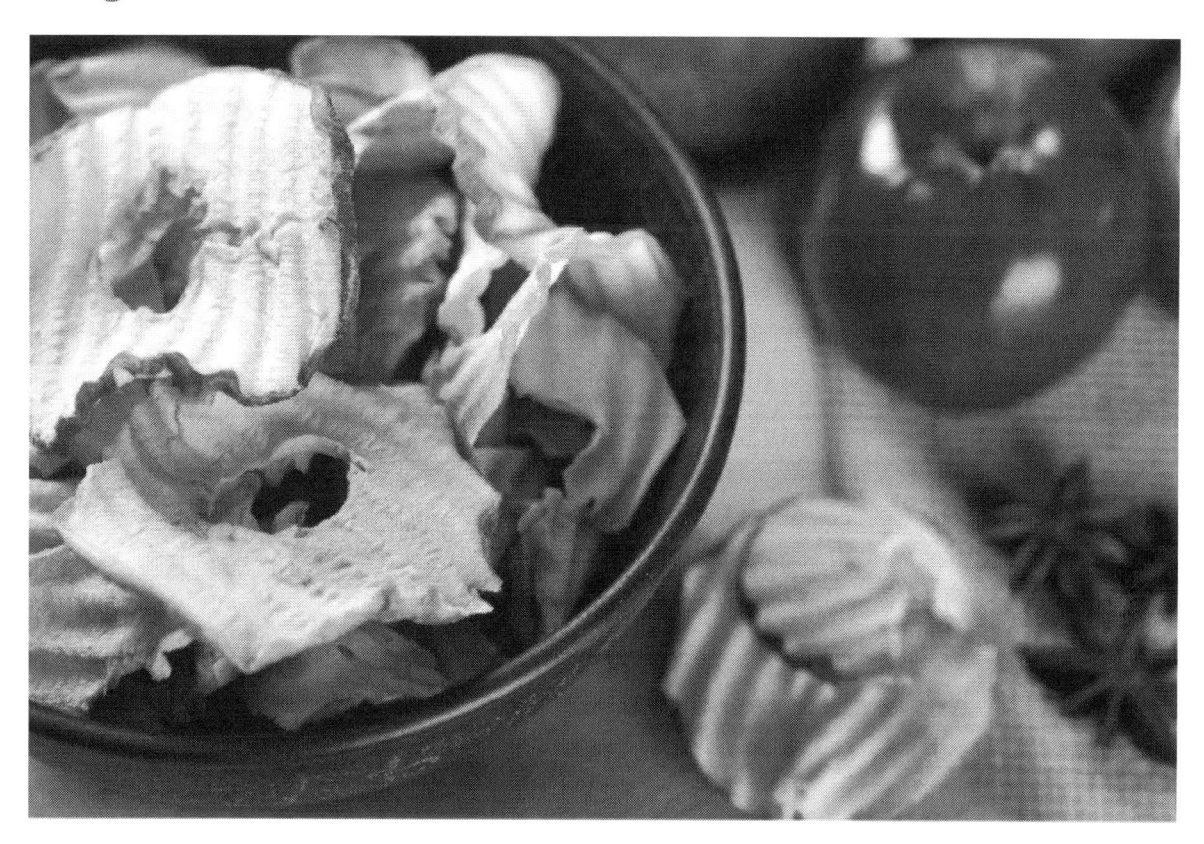

Ingredients:

- ➤ 4 large apples
- ➤ Ground cinnamon, to taste

Instructions:

1. Preheat the oven to 225°F and line two baking sheets with parchment.
2. Slice the apples as thinly as possible and arrange them on the baking sheet in a single layer.
3. Sprinkle with cinnamon then bake for 1 hour.
4. Flip the apple slices and let them cook for another hour.

5. Turn off the oven and let the slices cool until crisp then store in an airtight container.

Avocado Deviled Eggs

Servings: 6

Ingredients:

- 12 large eggs
- 2 small ripe avocadoes, pitted and chopped
- 2 tablespoons fresh lime juice
- 1 teaspoon garlic powder
- ½ teaspoon onion powder
- Salt and pepper to taste
- Paprika, to serve

Instructions:

1. Place the eggs in a saucepan and fill it with cold water.
2. Bring the water to boil then turn off the heat and cook the eggs, covered, for 10 to 12 minutes.
3. Transfer the eggs to an ice bath until they are cool enough to handle.
4. Peel the eggs and cut them in half lengthwise.
5. Scoop out the egg yolks and place them in a mixing bowl – arrange the egg halves on a serving tray.
6. Mash the egg yolks with the avocado, lime juice and spices.
7. Spoon or pipe the yolk mixture into the egg halves and sprinkle with paprika to serve.

Easy Coconut Flour Cupcakes

Servings: 12

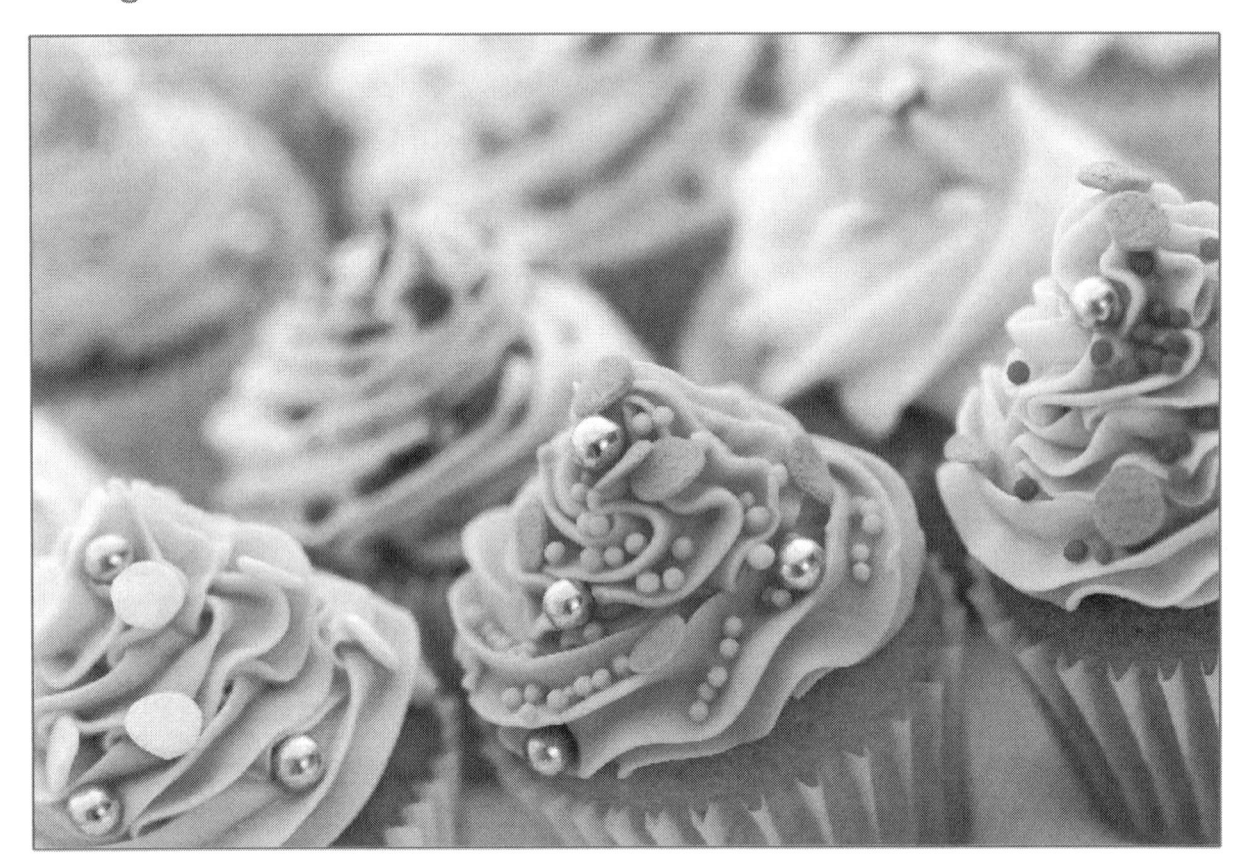

Ingredients:

- ½ cup sifted coconut flour
- ¼ teaspoon baking soda
- ¼ teaspoon salt
- 6 large eggs, whisked
- ½ cup coconut oil
- ¼ cup honey
- 1 tablespoon vanilla extract

Instructions:

1. Preheat the oven to 350°F and line a regular muffin pan with paper liners.
2. Combine the coconut flour, baking soda, and salt in a food processor.
3. Pulse several times then add the eggs, coconut oil, honey, and vanilla extract.
4. Blend smooth then divide the batter evenly in the pan.
5. Bake for 20 to 24 minutes until a knife inserted in the center comes out clean.
6. Cool the cupcakes for 1 hour then frost as desired.

Vanilla Almond Trail Mix

Servings: 8 to 10

Ingredients:

- 3 cups whole almonds
- 1 cup walnut halves
- 1 cup whole pecans
- 1 cup hulled pumpkin seeds
- 1 cup seedless raisins
- ¼ cup pure maple syrup
- ¼ cup melted coconut oil
- 1 teaspoon vanilla extract
- 1 teaspoon almond extract

Instructions:

1. Preheat the oven to 350°F and line a rimmed baking sheet with parchment.
2. Combine the nuts, seeds, and raisins in a large bowl.
3. In a separate bowl, whisk together the remaining ingredients.
4. Drizzle the wet mixture over the nuts and seeds then toss to coat.
5. Spread the mixture evenly on the prepared baking sheet.
6. Bake for 15 to 20 minutes until browned.
7. Let the trail mix cool completely then store in an airtight container.

Chocolate Chia Pudding

Servings: 4

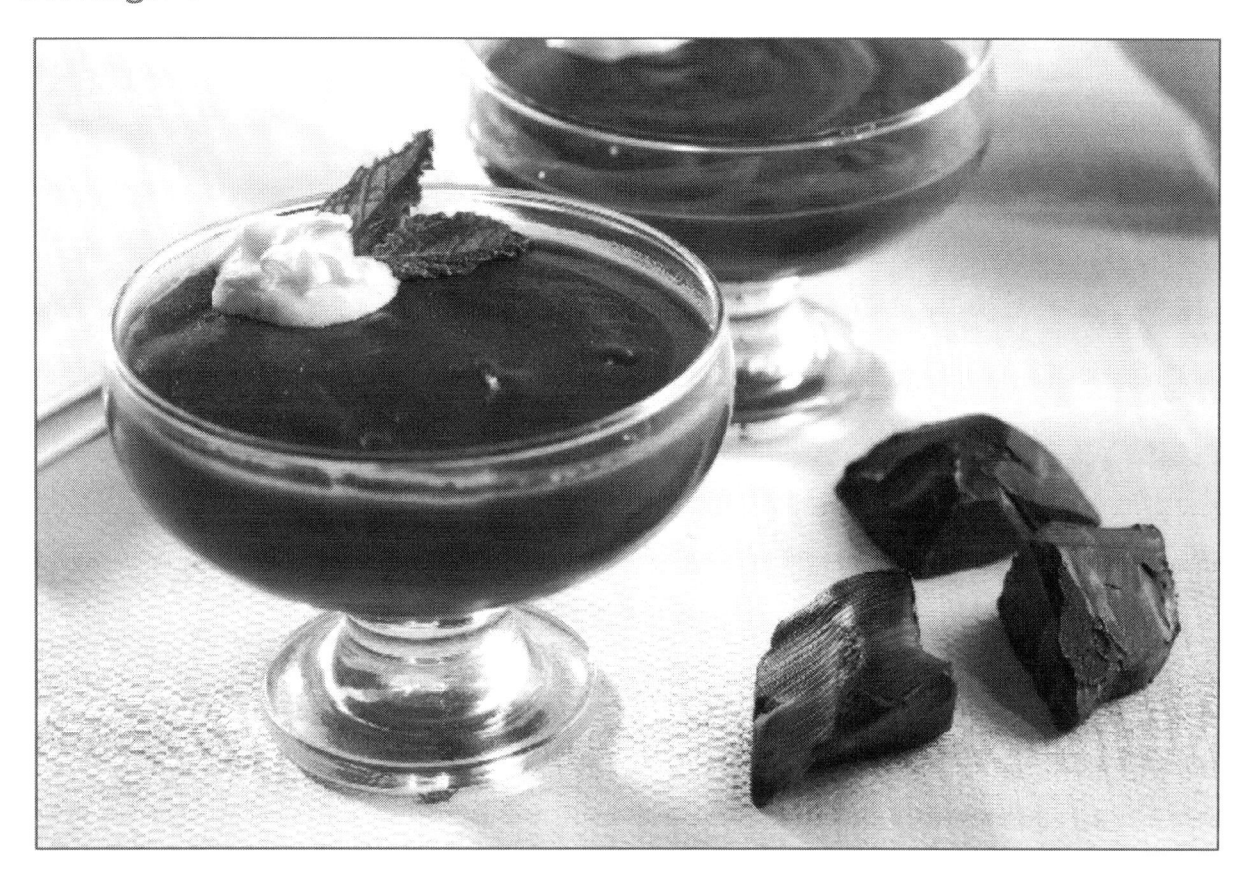

Ingredients:

- 1 ½ cups unsweetened almond milk
- 8 pitted Medjool dates
- ¼ cup unsweetened cocoa powder
- ¼ cup chia seeds
- 1 teaspoon vanilla extract

Instructions:

1. Combine the almond milk, dates, cocoa powder, chia seeds, and vanilla extract in a blender.

2. Blend on high speed for 30 to 60 seconds, scraping down the sides as needed, until smooth and well combined.

3. Spoon into dessert cups and chill until ready to serve.

Choco-Coconut Cupcakes

Servings: 12

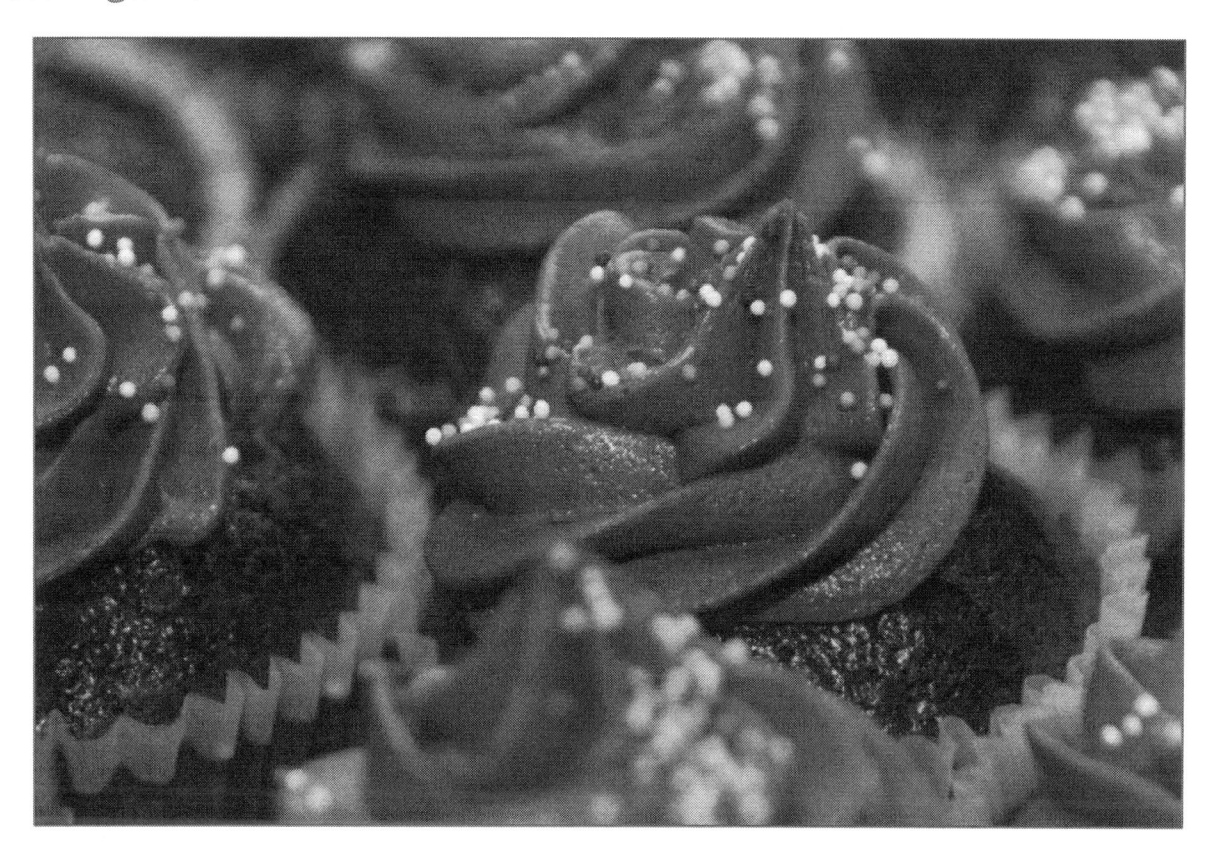

Ingredients:

- ¾ cup plus 2 tablespoons unsweetened cocoa powder
- ¾ cup almond flour
- 1 ½ teaspoons baking powder
- ¼ teaspoon salt
- 2/3 cup honey
- ½ cup unsweetened applesauce
- 2/3 cup coconut oil, melted
- 4 large eggs, whisked
- 2 tablespoons coconut sugar

- ➤ 2 teaspoons vanilla extract
- ➤ ½ cup shredded unsweetened coconut

Instructions:

1. Preheat the oven to 350°F and line the cups of a regular muffin pan with paper liners.
2. Combine the cocoa powder, almond flour, baking powder, and salt in a mixing bowl.
3. In another bowl, whisk together the honey, applesauce, and coconut oil until smooth.
4. Whisk in the eggs, coconut sugar, and vanilla extract.
5. Stir the dry mixture into the wet until it is just combined then stir in the coconut.
6. Divide the batter evenly among the cups and bake for 24 to 28 minutes until a knife inserted in the center comes out clean.
7. Cool the cupcakes for 5 minutes then remove to a wire rack to cool completely.
8. Frost as desired.

Sesame Kale Chips

Servings: 4 to 6

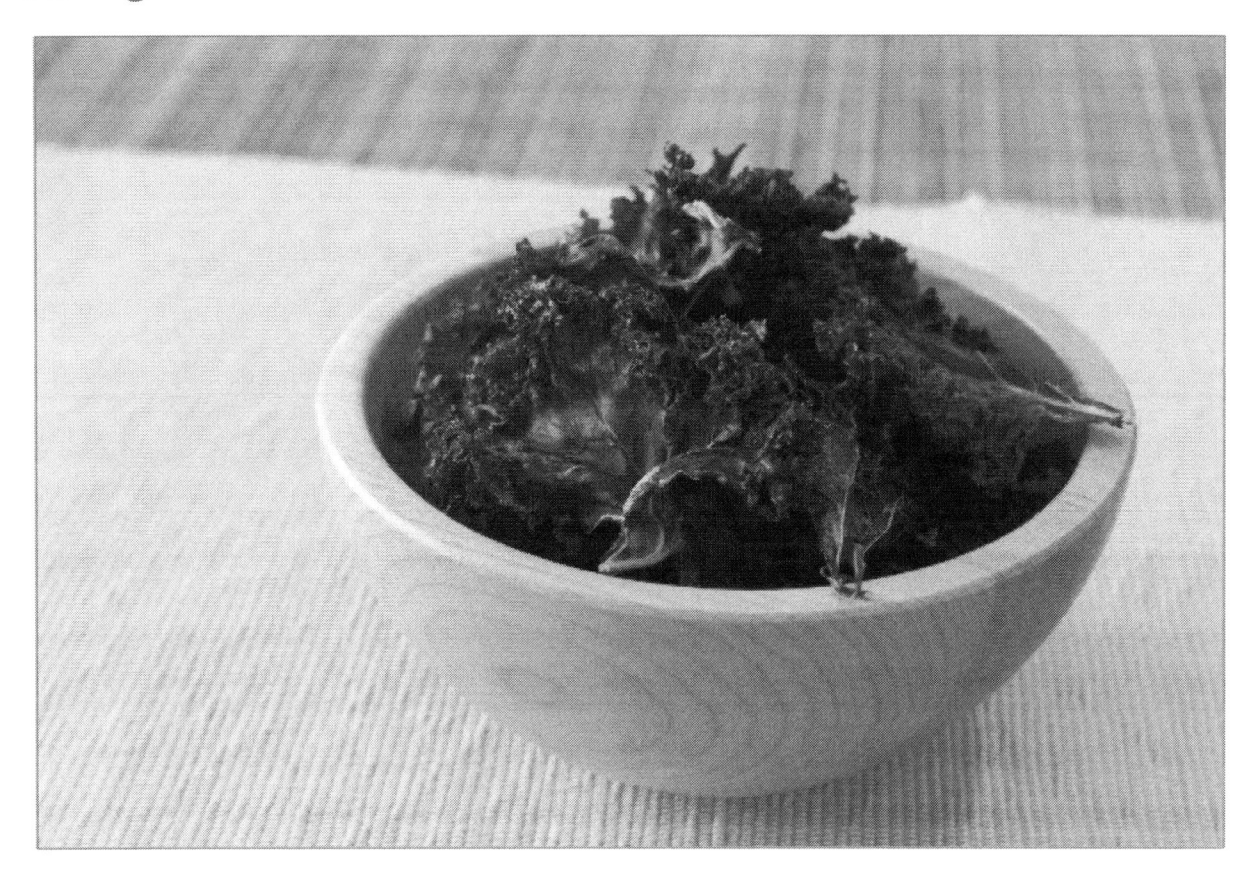

Ingredients:

- 2 large bunches of fresh kale
- Sesame oil, as needed
- Salt, as needed
- Sesame seeds, as needed

Instructions:

1. Preheat the oven to 350°F and line two baking sheets with parchment.
2. Trim the stems from the kale and cut the leaves into 2-inch pieces then arrange them on the baking sheet in a single layer.
3. Drizzle with oil and sprinkle with salt then bake for 12 minutes.

4. Sprinkle with sesame seeds then store in an airtight container.

Almond Butter Brownies

Servings: 8 to 10

Ingredients:

- 1 cup smooth almond butter
- 1/3 cup honey
- 1 large egg, whisked
- 2 tablespoons melted coconut oil
- 1 teaspoon vanilla extract
- 1/3 cup unsweetened cocoa powder
- ½ teaspoon baking soda

Instructions:

1. Preheat the oven to 325°F and grease a square baking pan.
2. Combine the almond butter, honey, egg, coconut oil, and vanilla extract in a mixing bowl.
3. Whisk until smooth and well combined.
4. Stir together the cocoa powder and baking soda in another bowl then stir the dry ingredients into the wet.
5. Spread the batter in the prepared pan and bake for 20 to 23 minutes until the brownies are set in the middle.
6. Cool the brownies completely before cutting to serve.

Cinnamon Roasted Nuts

Servings: 6 to 8

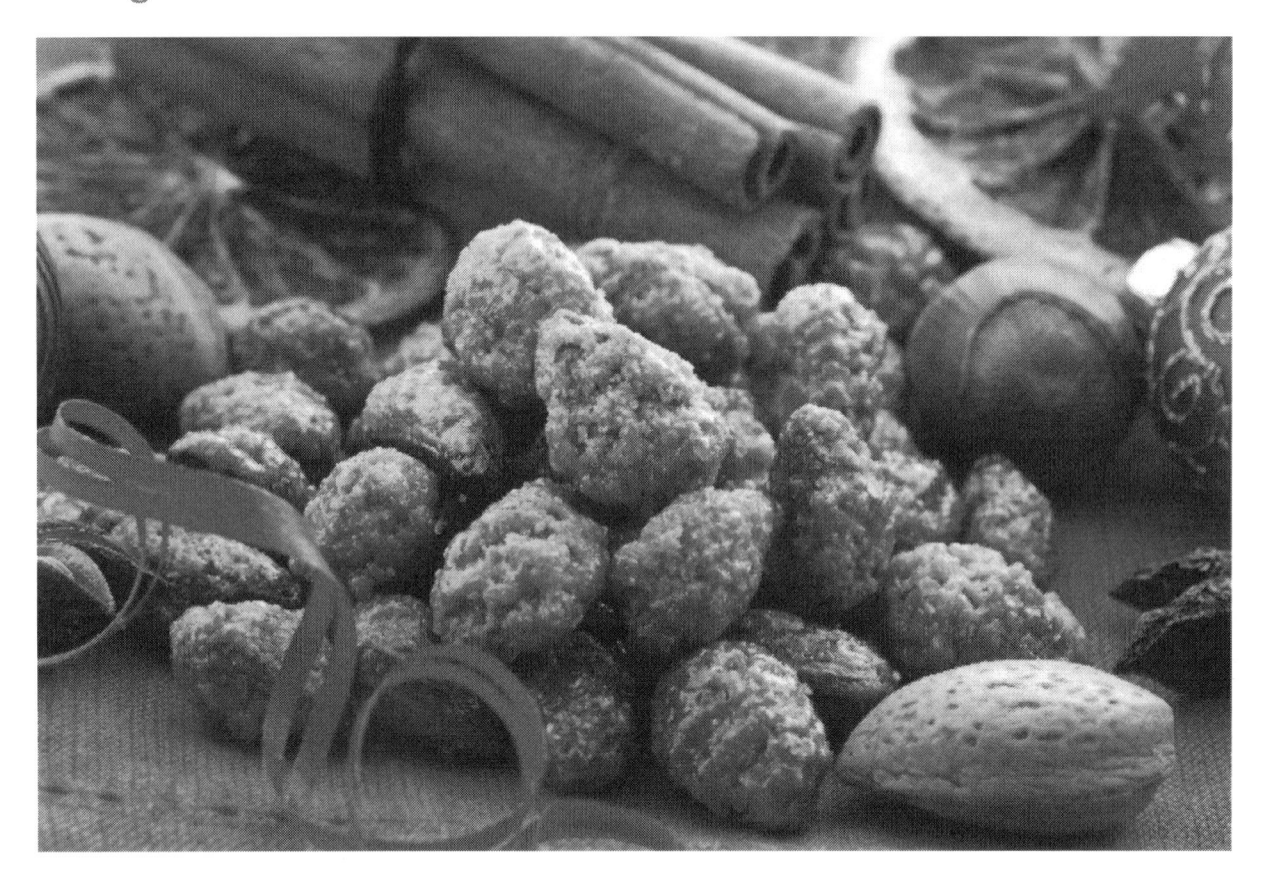

Ingredients:

- 2 cups whole almonds
- 2 to 3 teaspoons olive oil
- 1 teaspoon ground cinnamon
- ½ teaspoon salt

Instructions:

1. Preheat the oven to 250°F and line a baking sheet with parchment.
2. Place the almonds in a large bowl.
3. Add the olive oil, cinnamon, and salt then toss to coat.
4. Spread the almonds on the baking sheet and roast for 1 hour.

5. Remove from the oven and cool slightly to serve warm or cool completely and store in an airtight container.

Almond Flour Apple Crisp

Servings: 6 to 8

Ingredients:

- 2 pounds fresh apples, peeled and cored
- ¼ cup maple syrup
- 2 tablespoons orange juice
- 2 teaspoons ground cinnamon
- ½ teaspoon ground nutmeg
- ¼ teaspoon salt
- 1 ½ cups almond flour
- 2 tablespoons coconut oil, melted
- 1 tablespoon honey
- ½ teaspoon vanilla extract

Instructions:

1. Preheat the oven to 350°F.
2. Slice the apples very thin and spread them in a Dutch oven.
3. Stir in the maple syrup, orange juice, cinnamon, nutmeg, and salt.
4. Bring to a boil over medium-high heat then reduce heat and simmer, covered, for 8 to 10 minutes.
5. Make the topping by combining the almond flour, melted coconut oil, honey, and vanilla extract in a bowl.
6. Add a pinch of salt then stir until it forms a crumbled mixture.

7. Spread the apples in a glass baking dish and top with the crumbled mixture.

8. Bake for 20 minutes until the apples are hot and bubbling and the topping starts to brown.

Coconut Date Bites

Servings: 8

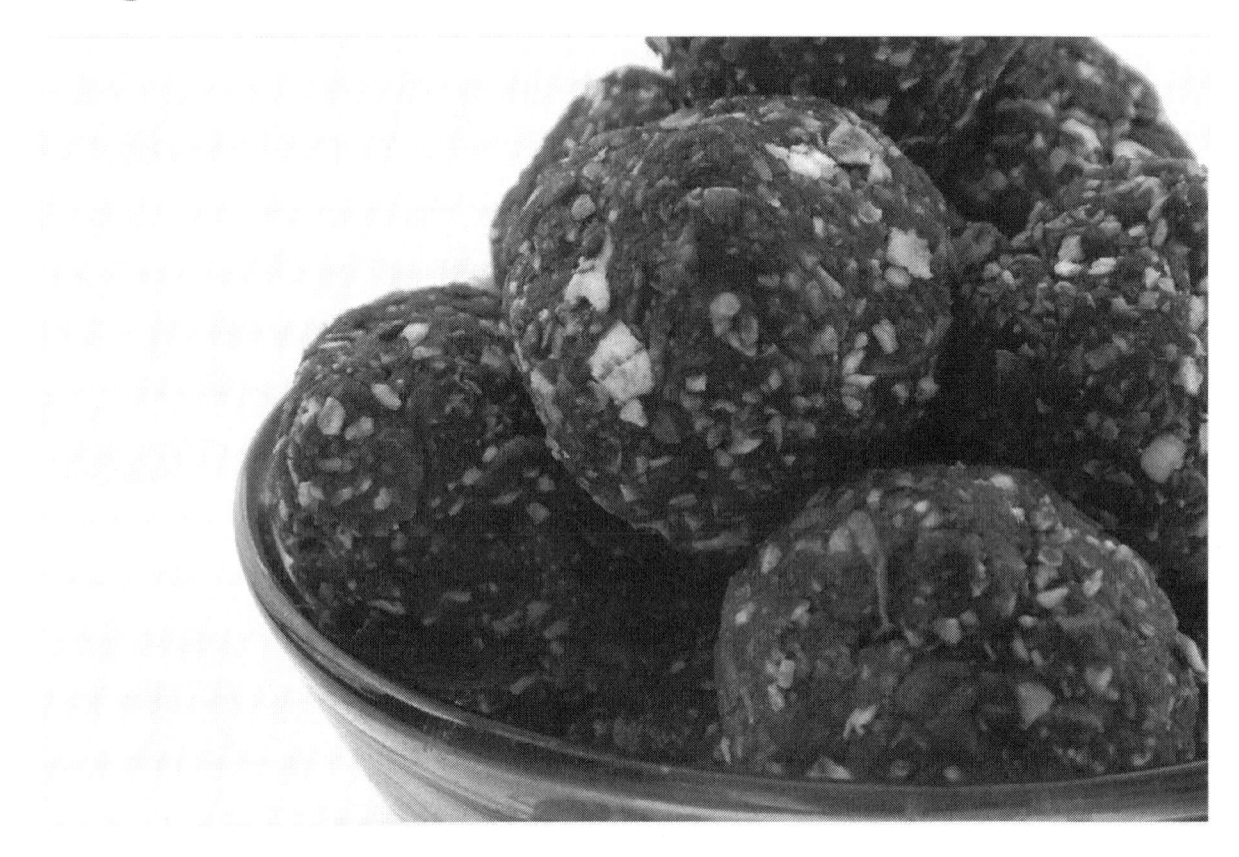

Ingredients:

- 1 cup raw honey
- ½ cup coconut oil
- 4 large eggs, beaten well
- 2 cups chopped pitted dates
- 1 ½ teaspoons vanilla extract
- 1 teaspoon salt
- 3 cups mixed chopped nuts
- 1 cup shredded unsweetened coconut

Instructions:

1. Whisk together the honey, coconut oil, and eggs in a medium saucepan over medium heat.
2. Stir in the chopped dates and bring to a boil.
3. Cook for 3 to 5 minutes, stirring occasionally, then remove from heat.
4. Stir in the vanilla extract and salt.
5. Add the nuts and coconut, then stir until well combined.
6. Shape the mixture into small balls by hand and arrange them on a plate.
7. Chill the coconut date bites until firm.

Lemon Blueberry Cupcakes

Servings: 12

Ingredients:

- ½ cup sifted coconut flour
- ¼ teaspoon baking soda
- ¼ teaspoon salt
- 6 large eggs, whisked
- ½ cup coconut oil
- ¼ cup honey
- 2 tablespoons lemon juice
- 1 tablespoon fresh lemon zest
- ½ cup fresh blueberries

Instructions:

1. Preheat the oven to 350°F and line a regular muffin pan with paper liners.
2. Combine the coconut flour, baking soda, and salt in a food processor.
3. Pulse several times then add the eggs, coconut oil, honey, lemon juice, and lemon zest.
4. Blend smooth then stir in the blueberries and divide the batter evenly in the pan.
5. Bake for 20 to 24 minutes until a knife inserted in the center comes out clean.
6. Cool the cupcakes for 1 hour then frost as desired.

Grilled Balsamic Peaches

Servings: 4

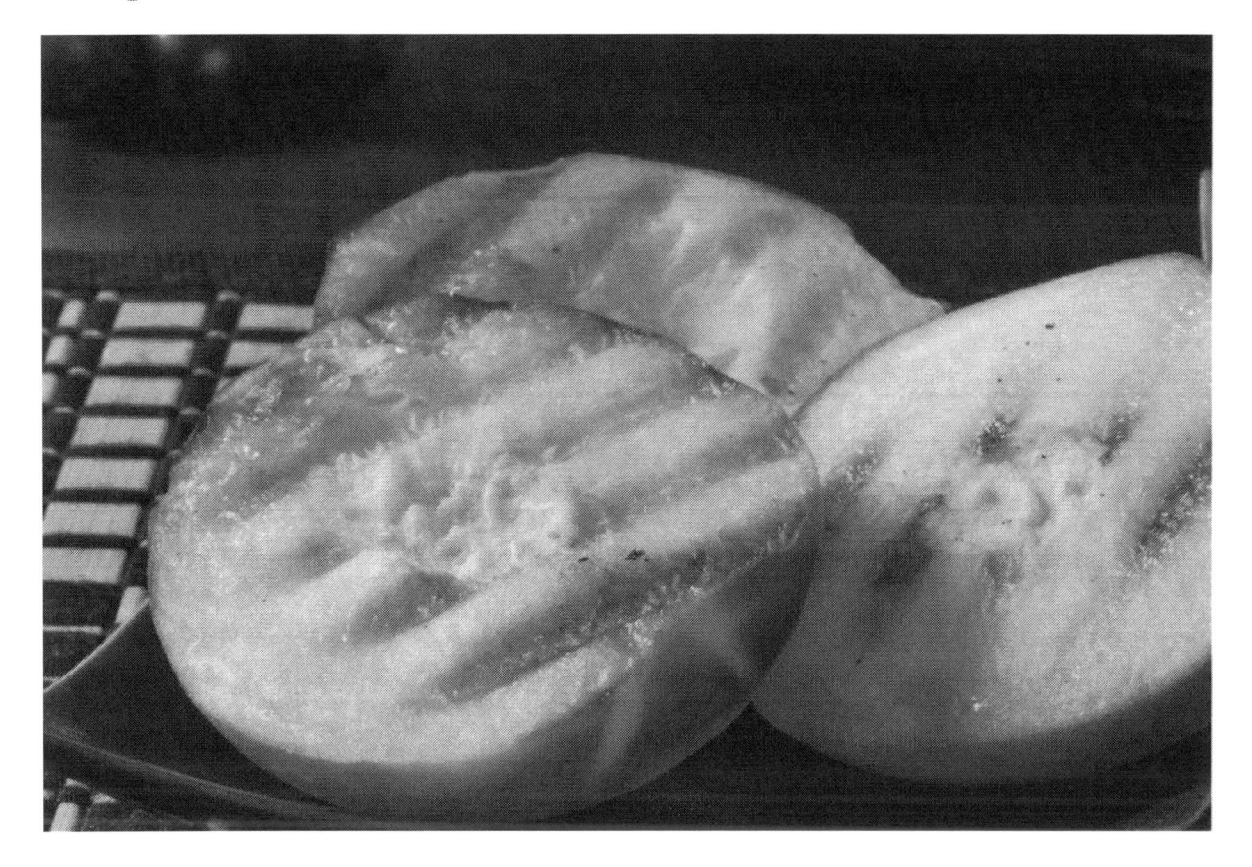

Ingredients:

- 4 ripe peaches
- Balsamic vinegar, as needed

Instructions:

1. Slice the peaches in half and remove the pits.
2. Preheat a grill pan to medium-low heat and spray with cooking spray.
3. Place the peaches cut-side-down on the grill and cook for 3 to 5 minutes until they just start to soften.
4. Transfer the grilled peaches to serving bowls and drizzle with balsamic vinegar to serve.

Maple Walnut Trail Mix

Servings: 8 to 10

Ingredients:

- 2 cups walnut halves
- 2 cups whole almonds
- 1 cup whole cashews
- 1 cup hulled sunflower seeds
- 1 cup seedless raisings
- ¼ cup pure maple syrup
- ¼ cup melted coconut oil
- 1 teaspoon almond extract
- 1 teaspoon ground cinnamon

Instructions:

1. Preheat the oven to 350°F and line a rimmed baking sheet with parchment.
2. Combine the nuts, seeds, and raisins in a large bowl.
3. In a separate bowl, whisk together the remaining ingredients.
4. Drizzle the wet mixture over the nuts and seeds then toss to coat.
5. Spread the mixture evenly on the prepared baking sheet.
6. Bake for 15 to 20 minutes until browned.
7. Let the trail mix cool completely then store in an airtight container.

Cinnamon Poached Pears

Servings: 4

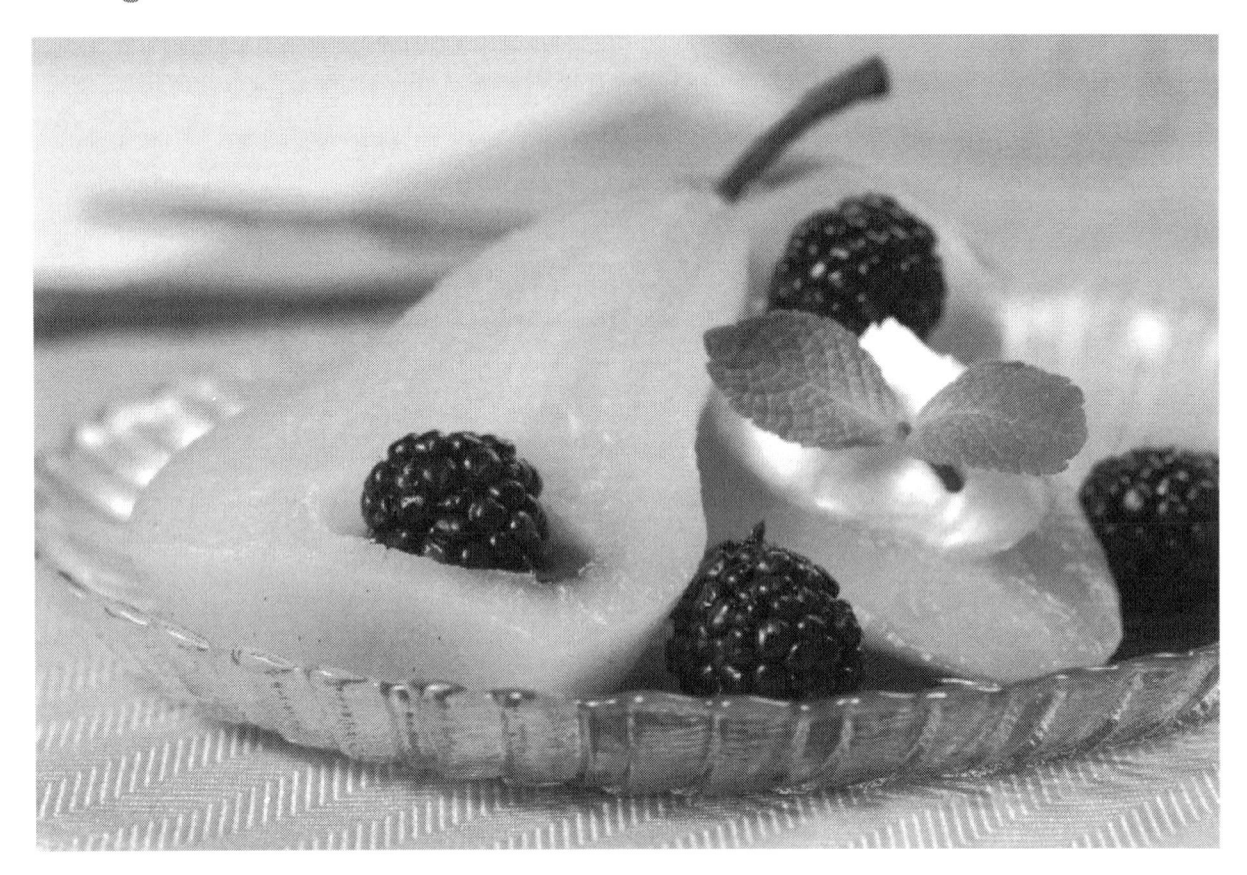

Ingredients:

- 4 large ripe pears
- 4 cups unsweetened cranberry juice
- ½ cup honey
- ¼ cup fresh squeezed orange juice
- 1 navel orange, sliced
- 2 cinnamon sticks

Instructions:

1. Whisk together the cranberry juice, honey, and orange juice in a large pot.

2. Add the oranges and cinnamon sticks and bring to a low boil.

3. Remove the cores from the pears and add them to the pot.

4. Simmer, covered, for 25 to 30 minutes until the pears are very tender.

5. Use a slotted spoon to remove the pears to serving bowls.

6. Drizzle with the poaching liquid, if desired, to serve.

Coconut Almond Chia Pudding

Servings: 3

Ingredients:

- 1 ½ cups unsweetened coconut milk
- 8 pitted Medjool dates
- ¼ cup unsweetened cocoa powder
- ¼ cup chia seeds
- 1 teaspoon almond extract

Instructions:

1. Combine the coconut milk, dates, cocoa powder, chia seeds, and almond extract in a blender.
2. Blend on high speed for 30 to 60 seconds, scraping down the sides as needed, until smooth and well combined.
3. Spoon into dessert cups and chill until ready to serve.

Baked Beet Chips

Servings: 4

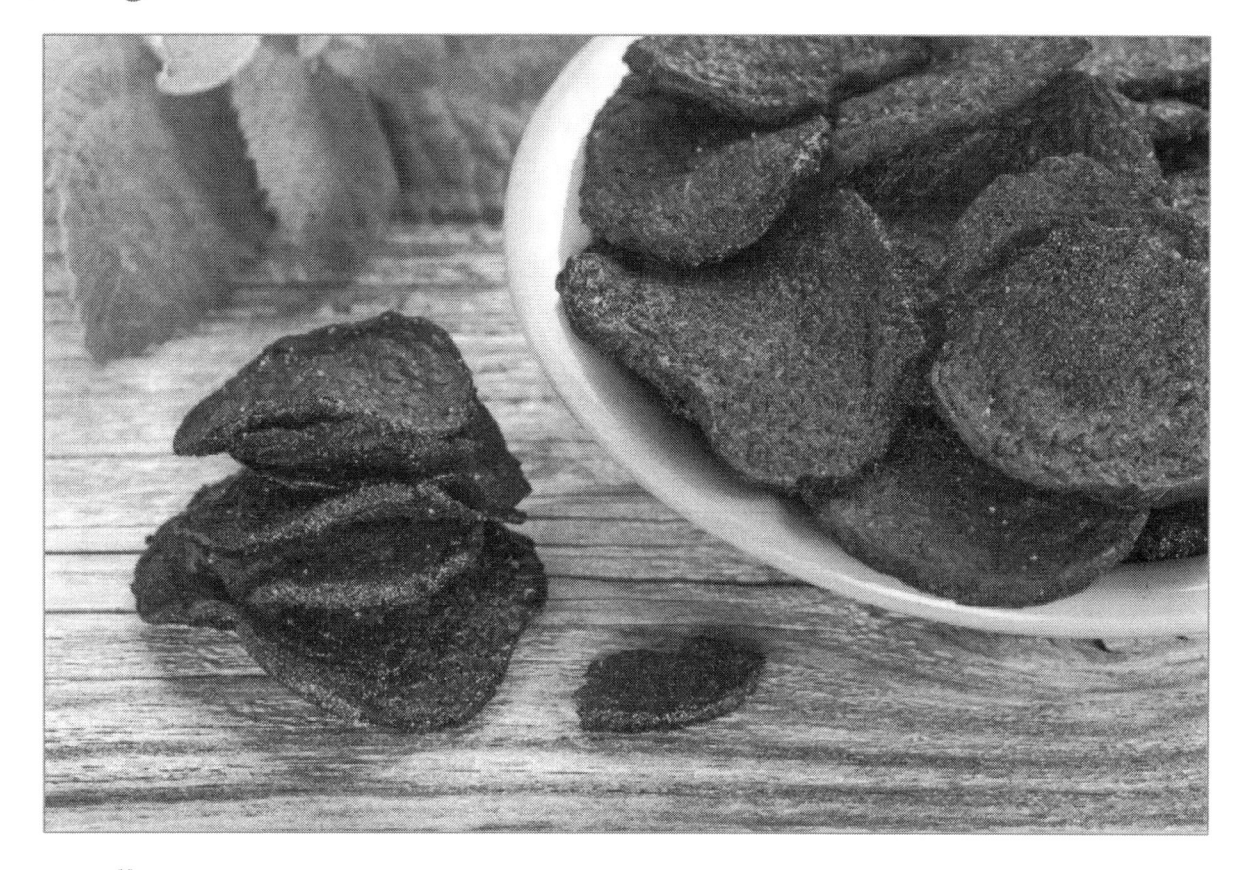

Ingredients:

- 5 whole beets, peeled
- Olive oil, as needed
- Salt and pepper

Instructions:

1. Preheat the oven to 175°F and line two baking sheets with parchment.
2. Slice the beets as thinly as possible and arrange them on the baking sheet in a single layer.
3. Drizzle with oil and season with salt and pepper then bake for 20 to 25 minutes, turning the tray halfway through.

4. Turn off the oven and let the slices cool until crisp then store in an airtight container.

Cranberry Coconut Trail Mix

Servings: 8 to 10

Ingredients:

- 2 cups whole cashews
- 1 cup walnut halves
- 1 cup whole pecans
- 1 cup whole almonds
- 1 cup shredded unsweetened coconut
- 1 cup dried cranberries
- ¼ cup pure maple syrup
- ¼ cup melted coconut oil
- 1 teaspoon vanilla extract
- 1 teaspoon ground cinnamon

Instructions:

1. Preheat the oven to 350°F and line a rimmed baking sheet with parchment.
2. Combine the nuts, seeds, coconut, and cranberries in a large bowl.
3. In a separate bowl, whisk together the remaining ingredients.
4. Drizzle the wet mixture over the nuts and seeds then toss to coat.
5. Spread the mixture evenly on the prepared baking sheet.
6. Bake for 15 to 20 minutes until browned.
7. Let the trail mix cool completely then store in an airtight container.

Bonus Content

Paleo Diabetic Protein Shakes

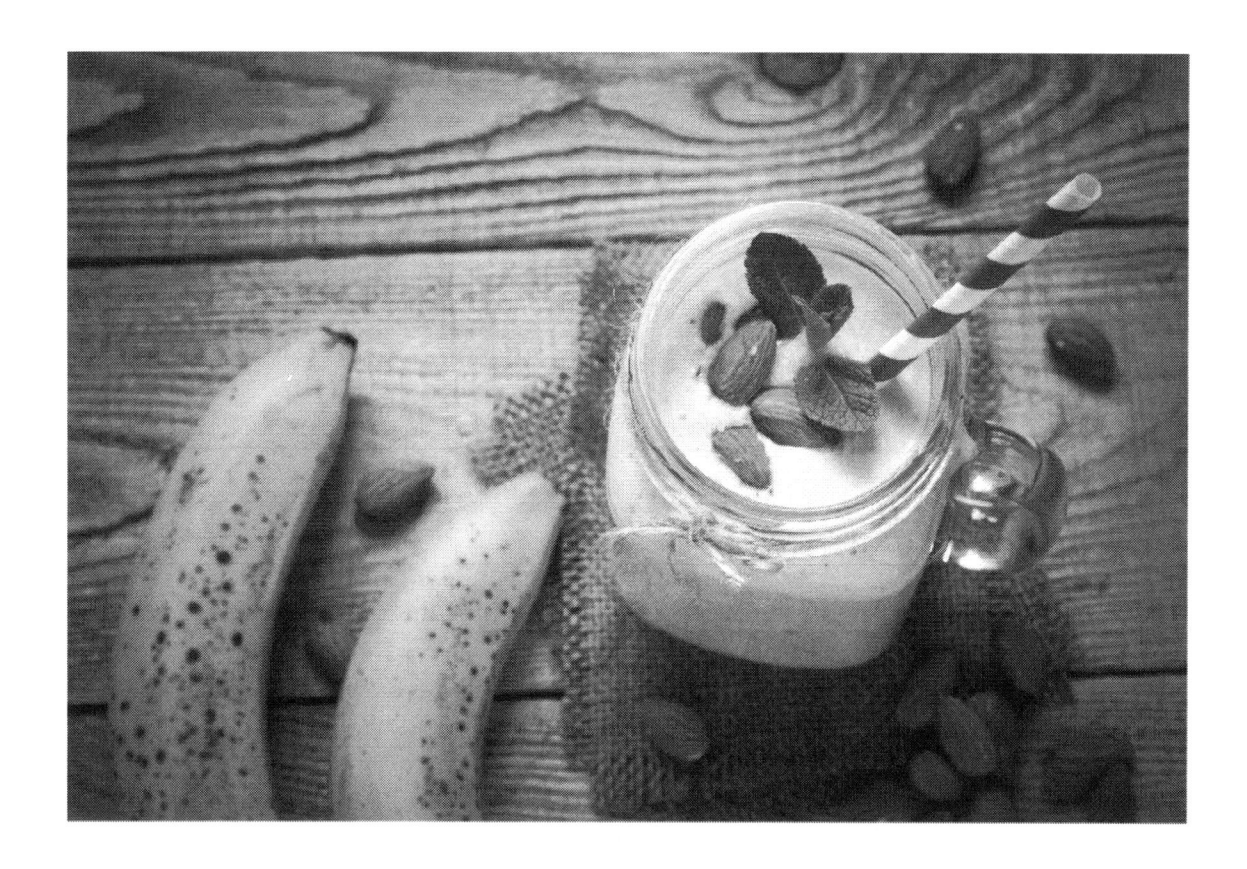

Recipes Included in this section		
Vanilla Almond Protein Shake	Chocolate Strawberry Protein Shake	Cinnamon Banana Protein Shake
Tropical Peach Protein Shake	Mocha Almond Protein Shake	Choco-Banana Coconut Protein Shake
Apple Pie Protein Shake	Brownie Batter Protein Shake	Almond Coconut Protein Shake
Coconut Cream Pie Protein Shake	Spiced Chai Protein Shake	Matcha Protein Shake

Vanilla Almond Protein Shake

Servings: 1

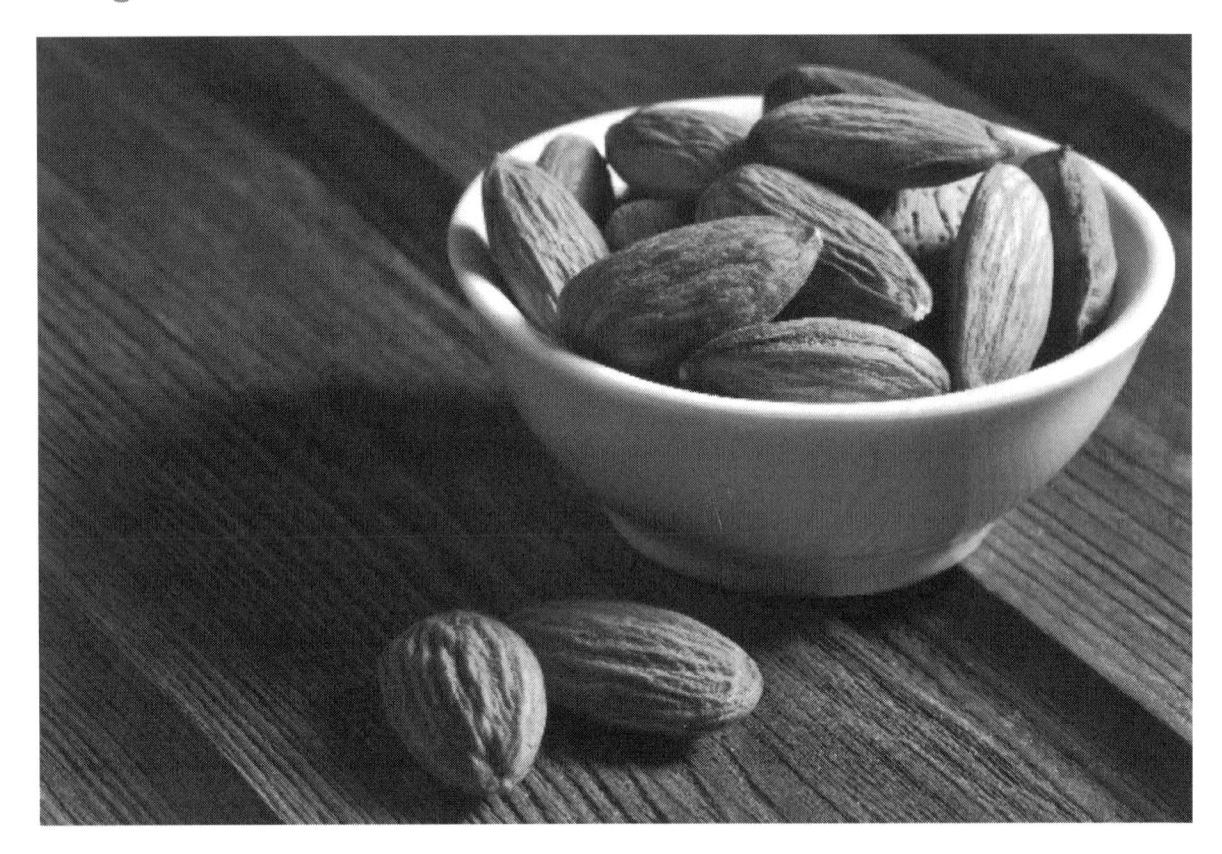

Ingredients:

- 1 cup unsweetened almond milk
- ¼ cup smooth almond butter
- 2 tablespoons vanilla hemp protein powder
- 1 tablespoon ground flaxseed
- 1 teaspoon honey
- 1 teaspoon vanilla extract
- Ice cubes, as needed

Instructions:

1. Combine the almond milk and almond butter in a blender.

2. Pulse the mixture several times then add the remaining ingredients.

3. Blend on high speed for 30 to 60 seconds until smooth.

4. Pour the protein shake into a glass and enjoy right away.

Chocolate Strawberry Protein Shake

Servings: 1

Ingredients:

- 1 ½ cups frozen sliced strawberries
- ½ cup unsweetened almond milk
- 2 tablespoons egg white protein powder
- 2 tablespoons canned coconut milk
- 1 tablespoon unsweetened cocoa powder
- 1 teaspoon honey

Instructions:

1. Combine the strawberries and almond milk in a blender.
2. Pulse the mixture several times to chop.
3. Add the remaining ingredients.
4. Blend on high speed for 30 to 60 seconds until smooth.
5. Pour the protein shake into a glass and enjoy right away.

Cinnamon Banana Protein Shake

Servings: 1

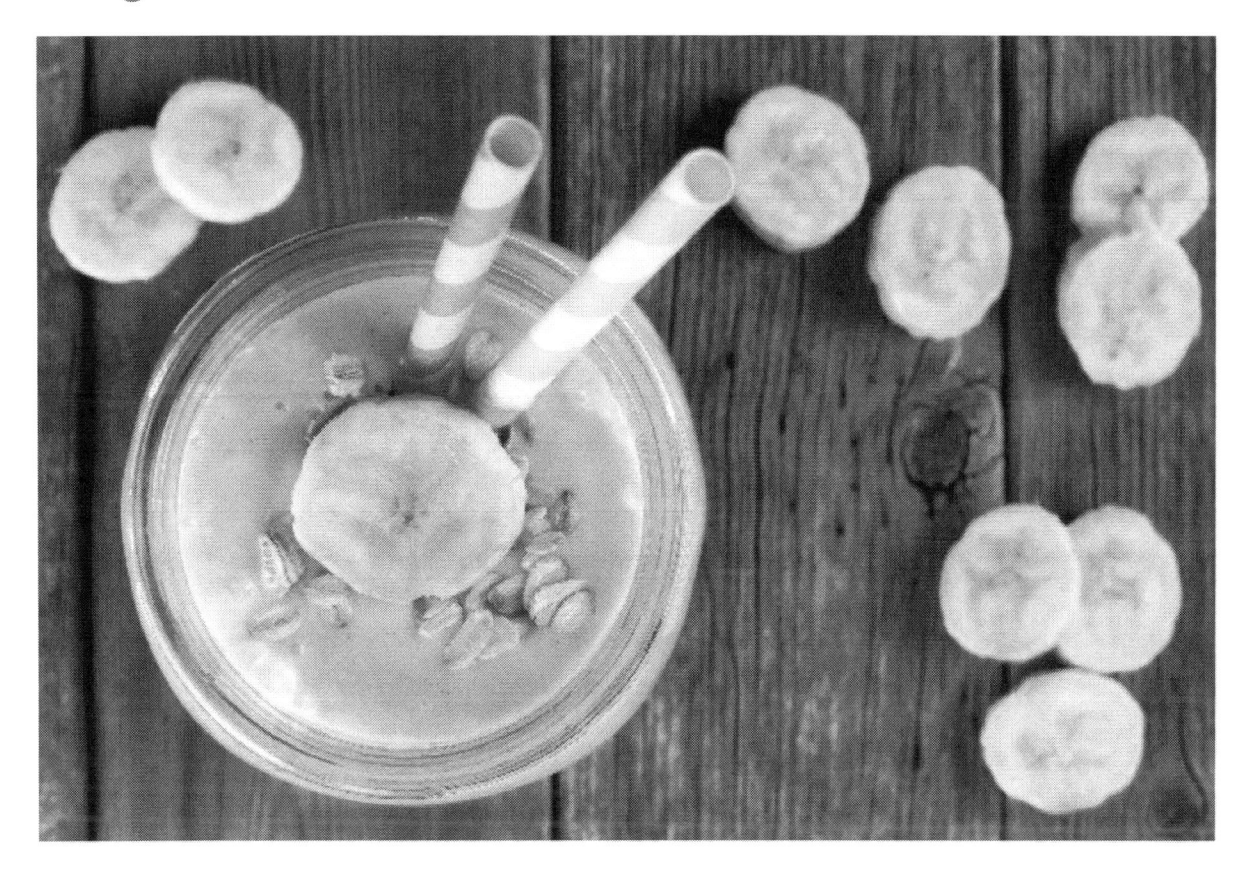

Ingredients:

- 1 large frozen banana, sliced
- ½ cup unsweetened almond milk
- ½ cup canned coconut milk
- 2 tablespoons almond butter
- 2 tablespoons hemp protein powder
- 1 teaspoon honey
- Pinch ground cinnamon

Instructions:

1. Combine the bananas and almond milk in a blender.

2. Pulse the mixture several times to chop.

3. Add the remaining ingredients.

4. Blend on high speed for 30 to 60 seconds until smooth.

5. Pour the protein shake into a glass and enjoy right away.

Tropical Peach Protein Shake

Servings: 1

Ingredients:

- 1 cup frozen sliced peaches
- 1 small frozen banana, sliced
- 1 fresh kiwi, peeled and sliced
- 1 cup unsweetened coconut milk beverage
- 1 cup ice cubes
- 1 teaspoon fresh lemon juice

Instructions:

1. Combine the peaches, bananas, and coconut milk in a blender.
2. Pulse the mixture several times to chop.
3. Add the remaining ingredients.
4. Blend on high speed for 30 to 60 seconds until smooth.
5. Pour the protein shake into a glass and enjoy right away.

Mocha Almond Protein Shake

Servings: 1

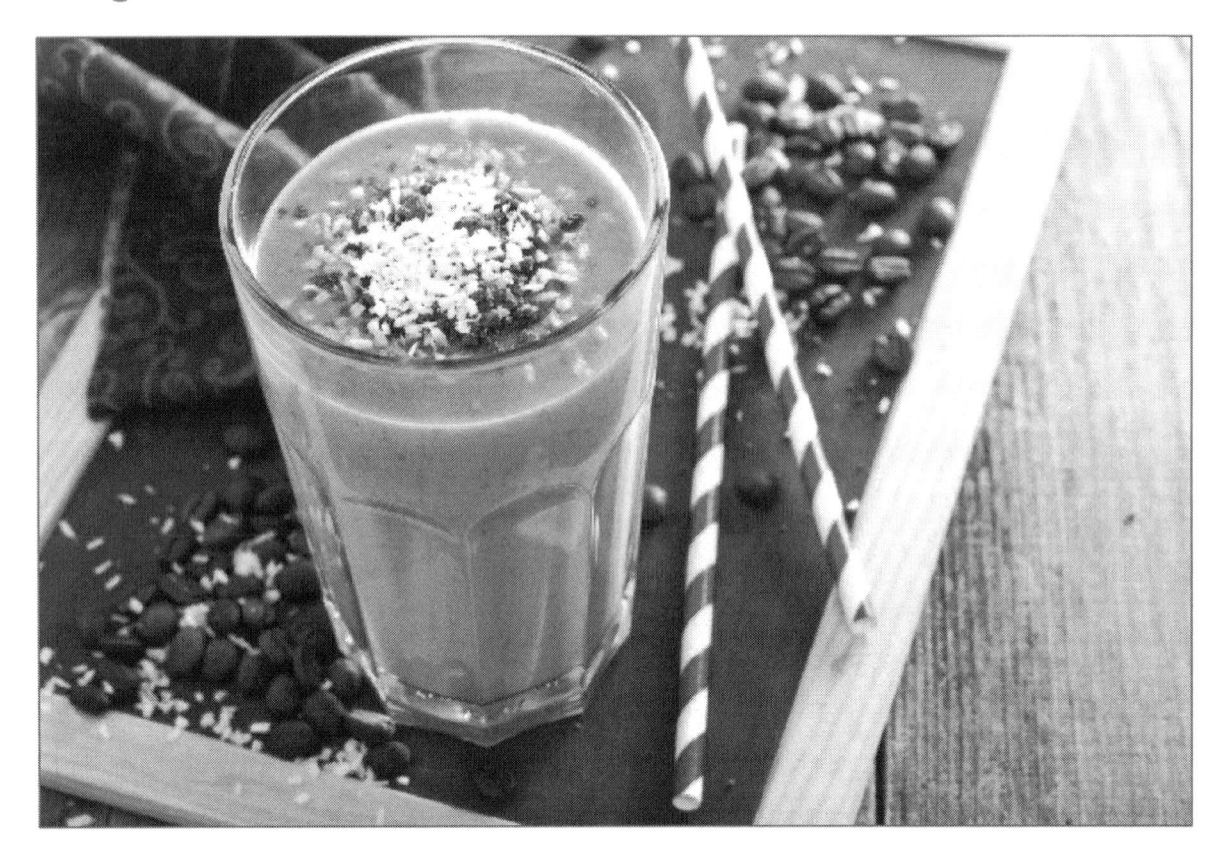

Ingredients:

- 1 large frozen banana, sliced
- ½ cup unsweetened almond milk
- ¼ cup canned coconut milk
- ¼ cup brewed coffee, chilled
- 1 tablespoon almond butter
- 1 teaspoon unsweetened cocoa powder
- Ice cubes, as needed

Instructions:

1. Combine the banana and almond milk in a blender.

2. Pulse the mixture several times to chop.

3. Add the remaining ingredients.

4. Blend on high speed for 30 to 60 seconds until smooth.

5. Pour the protein shake into a glass and enjoy right away.

Choco-Banana Coconut Protein Shake

Servings: 1

Ingredients:

- 1 large frozen banana, sliced
- 1 cup unsweetened coconut milk
- 2 tablespoons egg white protein powder
- 1 tablespoon unsweetened cocoa powder
- 1 tablespoon honey
- 1 teaspoon coconut oil
- ½ teaspoon vanilla extract

Instructions:

1. Combine the banana and coconut milk in a blender.
2. Pulse the mixture several times to chop.
3. Add the remaining ingredients.
4. Blend on high speed for 30 to 60 seconds until smooth.
5. Pour the protein shake into a glass and enjoy right away.

Apple Pie Protein Shake

Servings: 1

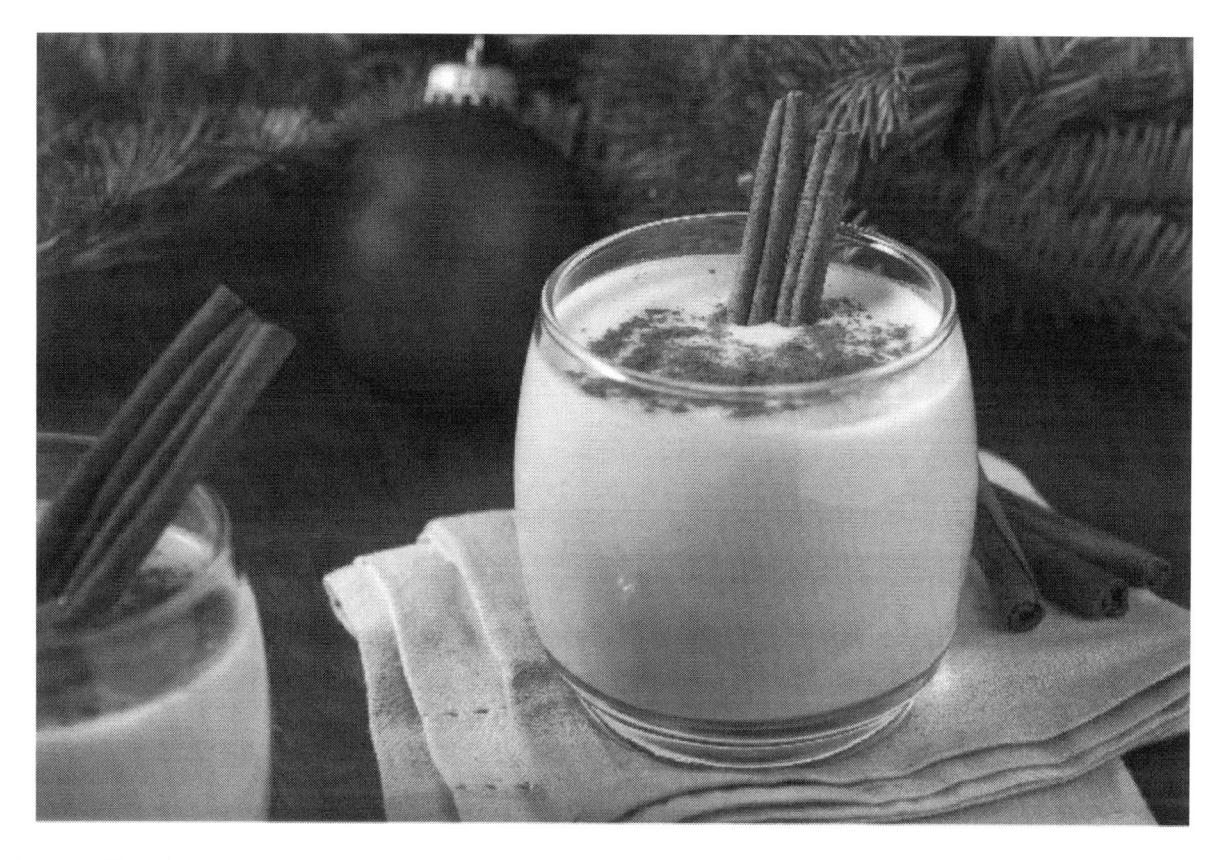

Ingredients:

- 1 small apple, peeled, cored, and chopped
- ¾ cup unsweetened almond milk
- ¼ cup chopped pitted dates
- 2 tablespoons hemp protein powder
- 1 tablespoon almond butter
- 1 teaspoon ground cinnamon
- Pinch ground nutmeg

Instructions:

1. Combine the apple and almond milk in a blender.

2. Pulse the mixture several times to chop.

3. Add the remaining ingredients.

4. Blend on high speed for 30 to 60 seconds until smooth.

5. Pour the protein shake into a glass and enjoy right away.

Brownie Batter Protein Shake

Servings: 1

Ingredients:

- 1 large frozen banana, sliced
- ½ ripe avocado, pitted and chopped
- 1 scoop egg white protein powder
- 2 tablespoons unsweetened cocoa powder
- ½ cup unsweetened almond milk
- ¼ cup canned coconut milk
- 1 teaspoon honey

Instructions:

1. Combine the banana, avocado, and almond milk in a blender.
2. Pulse the mixture several times to chop.
3. Add the remaining ingredients.
4. Blend on high speed for 30 to 60 seconds until smooth.
5. Pour the protein shake into a glass and enjoy right away.

Almond Coconut Protein Shake

Servings: 1

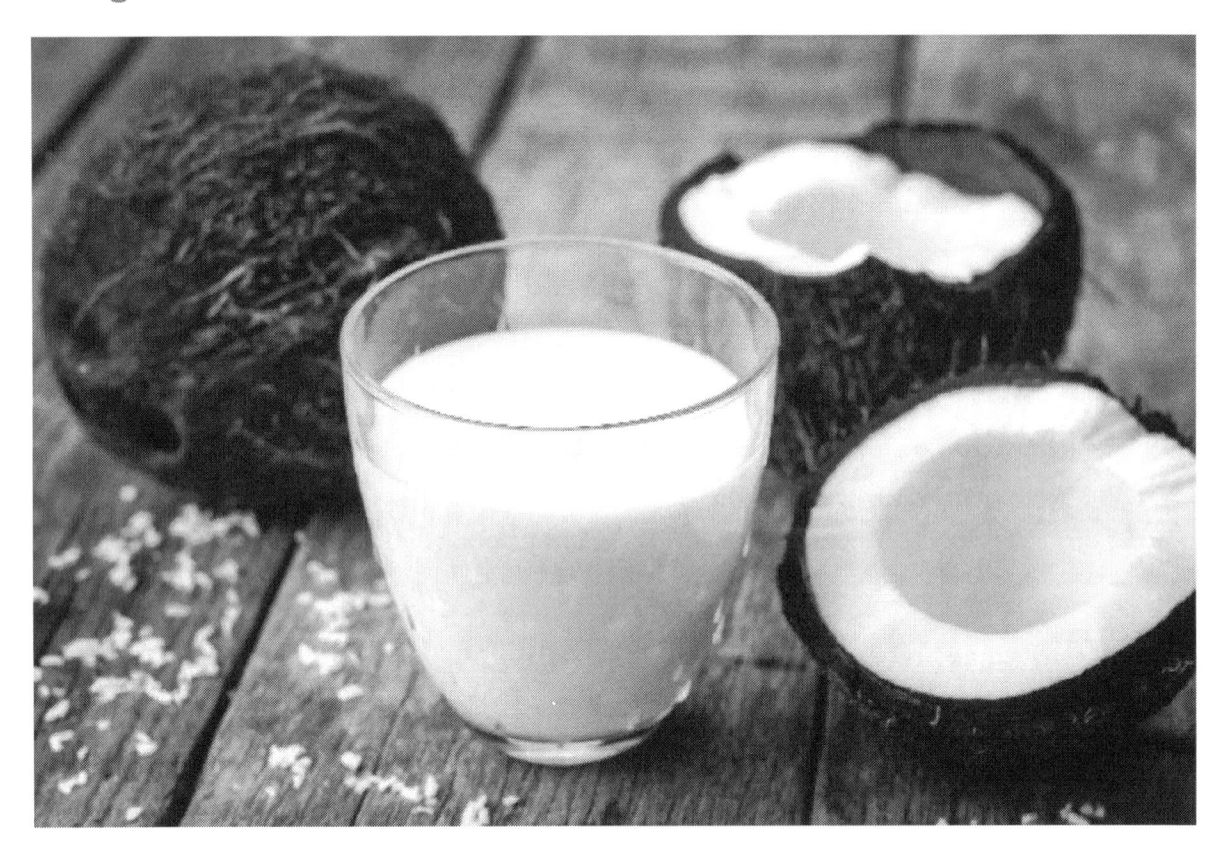

Ingredients:

- 1 small frozen banana, sliced
- ½ cup unsweetened almond milk
- ½ cup ice cubes
- 2 tablespoons hemp protein powder
- 2 tablespoons shredded unsweetened coconut
- 1 tablespoon sliced almonds
- 1 teaspoon honey

Instructions:

1. Combine the banana and almond milk in a blender.

2. Pulse the mixture several times to chop.

3. Add the remaining ingredients.

4. Blend on high speed for 30 to 60 seconds until smooth.

5. Pour the protein shake into a glass and enjoy right away.

Coconut Cream Pie Protein Shake

Servings: 1

Ingredients:

- 1 small frozen banana, sliced
- 1 cup light canned coconut milk
- ½ cup ice cubes
- 2 tablespoons hemp protein powder
- 2 tablespoons shredded unsweetened coconut
- 1 tablespoon honey

Instructions:

1. Combine the banana and coconut milk in a blender.
2. Pulse the mixture several times to chop.
3. Add the remaining ingredients.
4. Blend on high speed for 30 to 60 seconds until smooth.
5. Pour the protein shake into a glass and enjoy right away.

Spiced Chai Protein Shake

Servings: 1

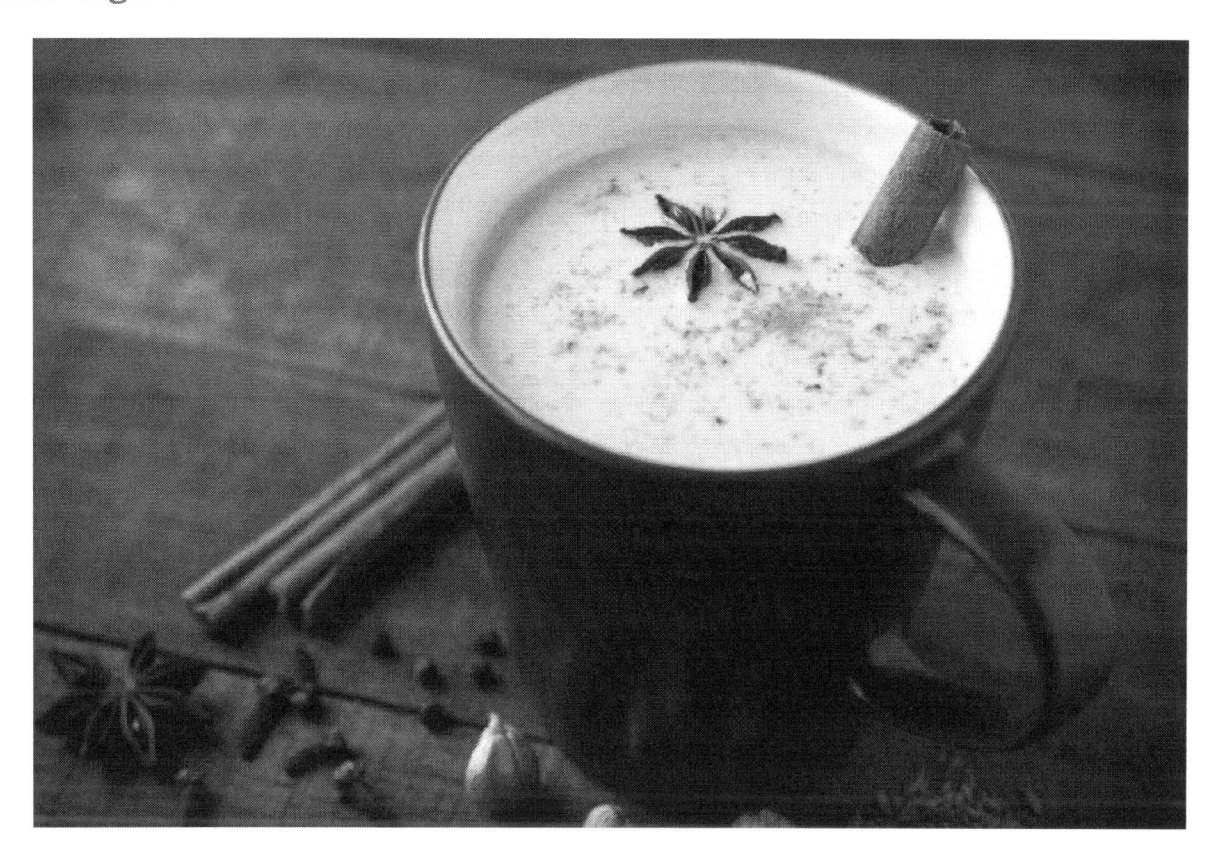

Ingredients:

- 1 small frozen banana, sliced
- 1 cup unsweetened almond milk
- 2 tablespoons hemp protein powder
- 1 tablespoon cashew butter
- 1 tablespoon ground flaxseed
- 1 teaspoon ground cinnamon
- ½ teaspoon cardamom
- ¼ teaspoon ground ginger
- Pinch ground cloves

Instructions:

1. Combine the banana and almond milk in a blender.
2. Pulse the mixture several times to chop.
3. Add the remaining ingredients.
4. Blend on high speed for 30 to 60 seconds until smooth.
5. Pour the protein shake into a glass and enjoy right away.

Matcha Protein Shake

Servings: 1

Ingredients:

- 1 small frozen banana, sliced
- ½ cup frozen chopped pineapple
- ½ cup chopped kale
- 1 cup unsweetened almond milk
- 1 tablespoon almond butter
- 2 teaspoons matcha powder
- 1 teaspoon chia seeds

Instructions:

1. Combine the banana, pineapple, and almond milk in a blender.
2. Pulse the mixture several times to chop.
3. Add the remaining ingredients.
4. Blend on high speed for 30 to 60 seconds until smooth.
5. Pour the protein shake into a glass and enjoy right away.

Conclusion

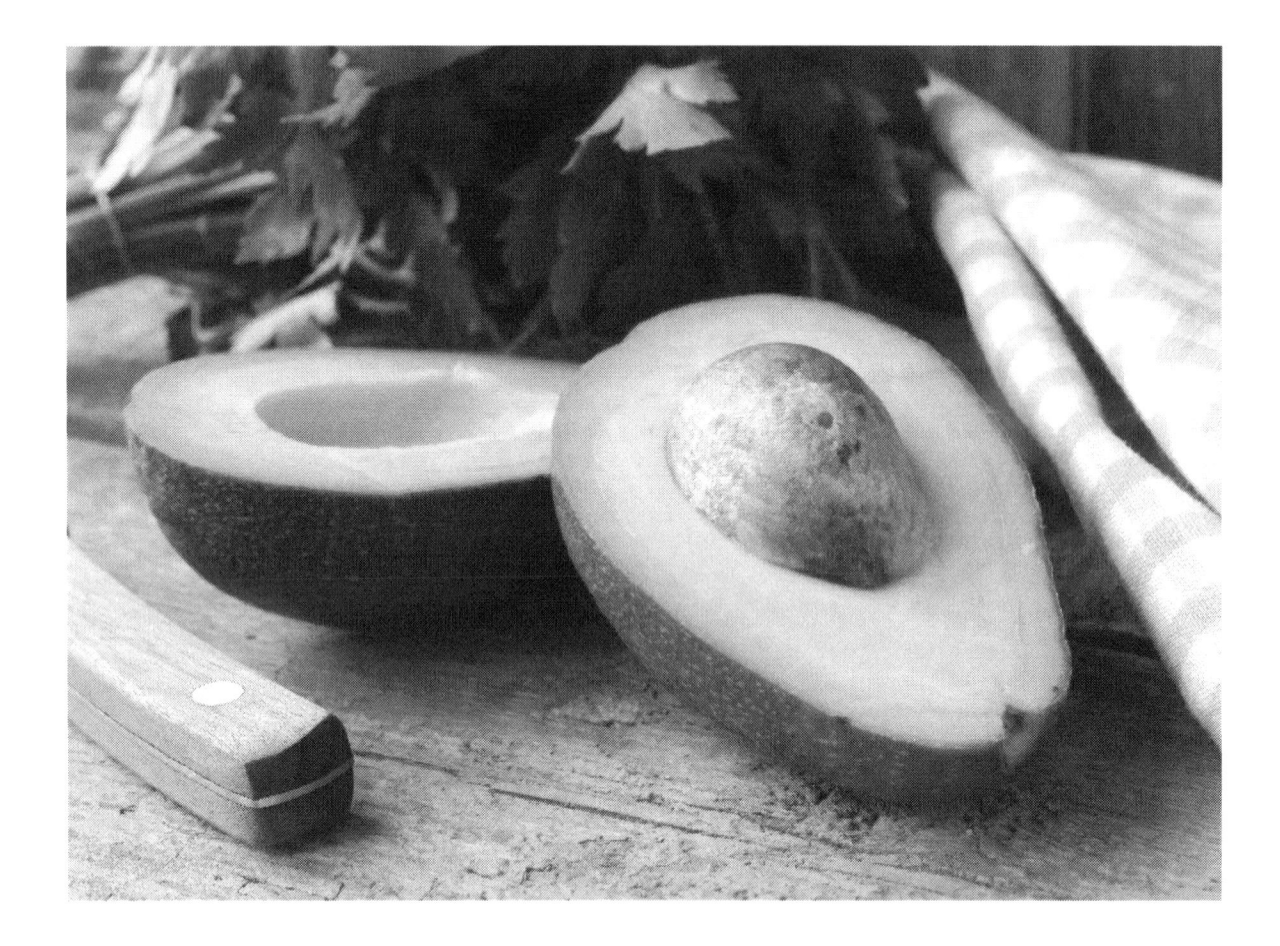

If you've been diagnosed with diabetes, it is up to you to take your health into your own hands. Making healthy changes to your diet and lifestyle can greatly improve your condition and, in the case of type 2 diabetes, may reverse it entirely. Keep in mind, however, that it takes time to make lasting changes so commit yourself to following the paleo diet and do your best to stick to it. The information provided in this book should help you to gain a comprehensive understanding of the diet as well as tips for getting started.

Diabetes is a serious condition that can lead to some pretty devastating consequences if left untreated. If you have diabetes, do yourself a favor and start getting it under control sooner than later. When you're ready to step up and make a change, follow the tips in this book and give some of the tasty paleo recipes a try!

The End

Thank you very much for taking the time to read this book. We sincerely hope you have gained something of value. We are here to serve you and every encouragement from you means a lot to us.

If you enjoyed this book, please be kind enough to review us and let us know what you liked about it or what you would love to see. This will help us produce better content for you guys and also help buyers out there make an informed decision when looking to make a purchase.

Made in the USA
Lexington, KY
25 September 2017